Baby & Me

The Essential Guide to Pregnancy

Third edition

Sixth printing, August 2000

Written by Deborah D. Stewart
Illustrated by Christine Thomas

Published by Bull Publishing Company

 This health education material has been reviewed favorably by the American Academy of Family Physicians Foundation.

To my daughter,
Christine,
who provided my inspiration.

The material in this publication is for general information only and is not intended to provide specific advice or recommendations for any individual. Your doctor or other health professional must be consulted for the advice with regard to your individual situation.

Copyright © 1997 Deborah Davis Stewart

Bull Publishing Co.
P.O. Box 208
Palo Alto, CA 94302
650-322-2855
www.bullpub.com

Third Edition, sixth printing, August 2000.

ISBN 0-923521-58-5

Library of Congress Catalog Card Number: 93-61740

CIP data available on request

Thank you...

First, to my beloved husband, Don Stewart, without whose imagination, encouragement, and patience this book would never have been born.

Second, to the rest of my family, Philip Davis, Mary Ellen Davis, Christine Richards, and Alex, who provided, in their own ways, constant support and belief in the importance of this effort.

Third, to my closest colleagues: Linda Ungerleider, R.N., M.S.N., A.C.C.E.; Steffie Goodman, M.S.N., C.N.M.; and Louise Roumagoux, M.S.N., M.P.H., whose hours of sharing ideas and editing were invaluable, especially for this third edition.

To Christine Thomas, who gave much more than just her inspired art to this project; to Kimberly Beba and Chung Ho Lee; and to the many other professionals and friends who contributed their support, thoughts, comments, and encouragement during the writing of this book.

Also, to the many reviewers in the medical and health insurance worlds whose critiques have made **Baby & Me** a better book. They include:

Reviewers of the Third Edition:

Marsha Frank, A.A.I., Account Manager, Acordia/Pettit Morry, Seattle, Washington;

Karma Metzgar, Nutrition Specialist, Life's Walk Community Coalition, St. Francis Hospital & Health Services, Maryville, Missouri;

Sheila Phelan, R.N., Humana Health Care Plans, Chicago, Illinois;

Lorna Seiler, R.N., C., Program Manager, MPower, ParaNatal Care of America, Edina, Minnesota;

Colina M. Stanton, R.D., L.D., Public Health Nutritionist, Central District Health, Valley County Office, McCall, Idaho;

M. Pamela Thompson, R.N., B.S.N., Allied Health Certification, Family Education Coordinator, Dept. of Obstetric Nursing, Massachusetts General Hospital, Boston, Massachusetts;

Donna Ugan, R.N., B.S., Director, Case Management, Gateway Health Management Services, Cleveland, Ohio;

Susan Wolcott, R.N., B.S.N., C.C.M., Manager of Case Management Services, Health Cost Consultants, Vienna, Virginia;

and...

Reviewers of the First Edition:

Richard S. Beamer, Vice President, Sedgewick, Noble & Lowndes, Seattle, Washington; Jerome Beekman, M.D., Chief of Staff, Group Health Cooperative of Puget Sound, Seattle, Washington; Arlene Erickson, Welfare Pension Administration, Seattle, Washington; Jeanne Fertado, Consultant, Godwins, Boone & Dickenson, Seattle, Washington; Michael Fleck, President, Pacific Health, Seattle, Washington; Vera Frinton, M.D., Vancouver, British Columbia, Canada; Donna J.H. Jensen, R.N.C., M.N., Prenatal Nurse Specialist, Nurse Manager, Family Beginnings, Group Health Cooperative of Puget Sound, Seattle, Washington; Florence Katz, Health Care Consultant, William M. Mercer, Inc., Seattle, Washington; Mary Jo Kraning, R.N., Manager, Northwest Hospital Childbirth Center (1983-90), Seattle, Washington; Nancy Magaña, M.S., R.D., C.D., Nutrition Consultant, Yakima Farmworkers' Clinic, Yakima, Washington; Greg McBride, C.C.D.C. III, N.C.A.C. II, Mental Health Counselor, Bellevue, Washington; K.C. McGowan, Executive Director/Consultant, Vitality Northwest, Edmonds, Washington; Diane McReynolds, Editor, *Personal Best*, Edmonds, Washington; Barbara J. Morrett, Vice President, Health Care Management, First Choice Network, Seattle, Washington; Jackie Oswald, Benefits Administration, Seattle, Washington; John Peterson, M.D., Seattle Heart Clinic, Seattle, Washington; David Pratt, M.D., Hershey Foods Corporation, Hershey, Pennsylvania; Peter Rabinowitz, M.D., Family Physician, Stamford, Connecticut; Sandra Randels, M.S.N., Coordinator, Fetal Alcohol Syndrome Program, Washington State Department of Health, Seattle, Washington; Mark Robinson, President, Wellness Solutions, Carrollton, Texas; Laurie Rosen-Ritt, M.Ed., Deaf Educator, Counselor for the hearing impaired at Planned Parenthood, Seattle, Washington; Annemarie Shelness, Child Passenger Safety Consultant, Sherman, Connecticut; Lynne Shepard, Residential Supervisor, Jericho Hills School for the Deaf, Vancouver, British Columbia, Canada; Karl Singer, M.D., Family Physician, Exeter Family Medicine Associates, Exeter, New Hampshire; Stephanie Tombrello, MSW, Executive Director, SafetyBeltSafe U.S.A., Los Angeles, California; William Trabold, Vice President, Fortis Benefits, Seattle, Washington; Linda Salsman Ungerleider, R.N., M.S.N., A.C.C.E., Assistant Professor in Nursing, North Park College, Illinois; James Weyand, M.D., Obstetrician, Group Health Cooperative of Puget Sound, Seattle, Washington; Mark D. Widome, M.D., Professor of Pediatrics, The Pennsylvania State University, Hershey, Pennsylvania; Two young women from Vancouver, British Columbia: one, hearing impaired; the other, a student of English as a second language.

I am also grateful to the Healthy Mothers, Healthy Babies Coalition of Washington State for the opportunity to write an earlier book on prenatal and infant care.

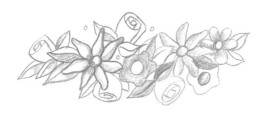

A message to you from me...

I know how much parents' health habits can affect a child. My baby—now a strong young woman—was a tiny premature infant 26 years ago. My husband, our families, and I all worried through her long stay in the hospital. We feared that she might have lasting health problems. If I had known many of the things I know now, she might not have been born so early.

I have written this book to give you the basic facts about staying healthy during pregnancy. The book will help you learn about pregnancy, birth, and caring for your new baby. It will also help you know what kinds of questions to ask to find out more.

The book also will help you enjoy this special time in your life. Your body is doing an amazing job. It has the power to grow and protect new life. Writing down what happens during your pregnancy could mean a lot to you later. Keep the book to remember this time after your baby grows up.

I hope *Baby & Me* will encourage you to do all you can for your child. Good health is one of the best gifts a parent can give a child. Caring for yourself and your baby is a big task. You deserve lots of help in making it easier.

Best wishes to you and your baby!

Deborah Davis Stewart
Seattle, Washington
May 1999

Table of Contents

Using this book

If you are already pregnant or planning to have a baby soon...

Taking care of yourself now is the most important thing you can do to have a healthy, happy baby. This book can help you do this. It can also help your baby's father understand what is happening to you. Share it with him.

- **The first three chapters** have basic information about taking good care of yourself and your unborn baby.

- **Chapters 4, 5, and 6** take you through your pregnancy, month by month.

- **Chapter 7** is about your baby's birth.

- **Chapter 8** gives you help in caring for your newborn baby.

- **The Purple Pages** is like the telephone "yellow pages." It has lists of useful organizations, services, and books that can give you more help during this time. A glossary gives you the meanings of words about pregnancy and health. An index helps you find what you want to know in this book.

This is one book you can write in as much as you like! Keep notes about how you feel and questions you want to remember to ask your doctor, nurse, or nurse-midwife at your next checkup. Record pages give you places to note when you first feel your baby kick or hear his or her heart beating. You will enjoy looking back at these pages and remembering this special time.

Now is a good time to take a quick look all the way through the book. Keep it where you can find it easily. I hope you will use it often.

Family or ethnic health habits

Health habits and advice in this book may be different from what your own family or your people have done in the past. For example, in some cultures, certain foods are not eaten during pregnancy. In others, the baby's father may not take part in the birth.

There are many ways to good health. The ideas in this book will give you and your baby a good chance for a healthy start. **If your ways are different, talk about them with your doctor, nurse, or nurse-midwife.**

Special words

Because some babies are girls and some are boys, I take turns using "he" and "she" to mean any baby. In the same way, I may use "she" or "he" to refer to a doctor, nurse, or nurse-midwife.

I have used the words "health care provider" or "provider" in some places to mean your doctor, nurse-midwife, or nurse.

I have tried to use as few long medical words as possible. You may want to learn the ones you read here, because your doctor or nurse-midwife will probably use them. You will find their meanings on the page where they first appear. When you see a word marked like this (*), look for its definition at the side of the page. The definitions are also in the glossary at the back of the book.

> ***Please note:*** *This book should not be the only guide you use to care for yourself and your unborn child. Your doctor or nurse-midwife is trained to help you take care of your own special needs.*

Memories of Pregnancy

This page is for keeping notes on things you want to remember about your pregnancy. There is a page for birth notes at the end of Chapter 7.

Date when I found out I was pregnant

_____

What I was doing the day I found out I was pregnant

_____

_____

Nickname I called my unborn baby

_____

When I heard my baby's heart beat for the first time
_____ (date)

How I felt _____

_____

Baby's first hiccup _____ (date)

What it felt like_____

_____

Baby's first kick _____ (date)

Day or night? _____

What it felt like _____

_____

My first contractions _____ (date)

What did they feel like? _____

_____

Chapter 1

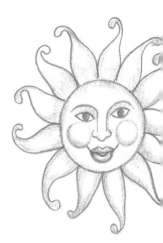

Get Ready for Pregnancy

Are you having sex?

Are you planning to have a baby?

Do you think you might be pregnant?

Are you already expecting?

Women often get pregnant when they are not planning to have a baby. **So it is never too soon to make your body a healthy home for your baby.**

Before you get pregnant is the best time to make sure your body is ready. But if you are already pregnant, start now. This way, your unborn baby will have a safe place to grow.

Most babies are born healthy, but some are born with health problems. Some problems begin before a woman knows she is pregnant. Others happen as the baby grows. A woman's health also can be affected by pregnancy.

Some problems can be prevented. Many others can be made less serious. Preventing a problem now is better than trying to fix it later. One problem that often can be prevented is preterm birth, when a baby is born too early.

What you do now is important for your baby's health—and your own.

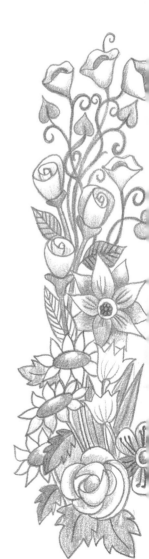

What every mother-to-be needs to know

Plan to get pregnant when you are ready to care for a baby. You and your child will both have a better life when you are healthy, happy, and able to pay the costs of raising a child.

Your age is important. Many pregnant teens face difficulties with health, money, and education. Some women who get pregnant after age 40 have added health problems. Also, their babies have a greater risk of birth defects. Talk with your health care provider if your age worries you.

Whatever age you may be, you can prepare your body to be a healthy home for an unborn child. **The most important things you can do before and during pregnancy are:**

- **Live a healthy life and stop unhealthy habits.** (See page 14 and Chapter 2 for more about this.)

- **Learn about pregnancy**, birth, and parenting. Use this book. Ask questions about things you do not understand.

- **Get health care now**. Before you get pregnant, take care of any health problems you have. Once you are pregnant, get regular prenatal checkups. Be sure to follow medical advice.

- **Share your joys and your worries** with your husband or partner and friends.

Your habits, your health, and your family's health history can affect your baby. Look at the list on the next page for some of the things that could lead to problems.

■ ■ ■ ■ ■ ■ ■ ■ ■ ■

Tip–Paying for care: Find out how your prenatal health care will be paid for. Discuss this with your insurer, employee benefits office, or clinic. How much will be covered? What will you have to pay yourself?

Check your health history

The items below could give you problems during pregnancy or cause your baby to be born too early. Knowing about them now, you can do everything possible to keep yourself and your baby healthy.

Check the items below that are true for you.

Yes (✔)

____ I often do not eat fruits or vegetables three times a day.

____ I think I am too fat or too thin and diet often.

____ I smoke cigarettes.

____ I drink more than one glass of beer, wine, wine cooler, or hard liquor each week.

____ I take medicines often.

____ I have used illegal drugs.

____ I am exposed to X-rays, dangerous chemicals, or lead at work.

____ I have diabetes, seizures, or high blood pressure.

____ I have had infections in my vagina that were hard to cure.

____ I have or have had an STD,* like herpes, chlamydia, gonorrhea, syphilis, or HIV/AIDS.

____ I am younger than 18 or older than 34.

____ I have had problems during a pregnancy or have had a baby who weighed less than $5\frac{1}{2}$ pounds at birth.

____ I have had a miscarriage.

____ Someone in my family has had a serious birth defect or problems during pregnancy.

____ A family member has an illness that is passed from parent to child, like cystic fibrosis, hemophilia, sickle cell disease, or Tay-Sachs disease.

*STD: A sexually transmitted disease, that is passed from one person to another when they have sex.

Tell your health care provider about the items you have checked. Learn how they could affect your baby. Many of them can be stopped or corrected. **What you do can make a difference!**

Healthy habits before pregnancy

Many pregnancies are a surprise. If you are having sex, you could get pregnant. That's why it is so important to change your habits now.

Important parts of your baby's body start to grow soon after conception.* Anything that harms the tiny embryo* at this time can do serious damage before you know you are pregnant. For this reason, **make sure your body is healthy before you get pregnant.**

*Conception: The beginning of a baby's growth, when the mother's egg unites with the father's sperm.

*Embryo: The word used for the unborn baby in the first 8 weeks after conception. After that time, it is called a fetus.

Steps to take

✔ **Get any health problems under control**. Conditions like diabetes and high blood pressure can affect your pregnancy.

✔ **Stop using alcohol, tobacco, and any illegal drugs.** Any time you smoke, drink alcohol, or use street drugs, your baby gets a dose, too. If you have trouble stopping, ask for help. You can quit!

✔ **Ask your health care provider about the effect of any medicines you take on an unborn baby.** Many medicines used for colds, headaches, or dieting can do harm. Even some prescription drugs can affect your baby.

✔ **Get your body weight to a healthy level.** If you are too thin, your baby could be born early. If you are too heavy, your baby's health and your own could be in danger. A dietician could help you.

✔ **Take a vitamin pill every day and eat healthy foods.** Every woman needs to get enough folic acid every day. (See the next page.) Your body needs plenty of milk, fruits, vegetables, whole grains, and water. This is a good time to learn healthy eating habits. (See pages 34 through 40.)

✔ **Talk with your partner** about your wish to have a baby. Make sure you have his support before you get pregnant.

Protect your baby's fragile body

The brain and spinal cord* are the most important parts of a person's nervous system. They control how you think and move. They begin to grow in the first few weeks of life. It is easy to damage them without intending to.

You can help prevent brain and spinal cord problems. **You must do these things before you get pregnant**.

Avoid alcohol, cigarettes, and other drugs

Beer, wine, and hard liquor affect the growth of a baby's brain. Alcohol is the main cause of mental retardation. Even one drink could cause harm. You can prevent this damage by not drinking.

Cigarette use slows an unborn baby's growth. It can lead to preterm birth.* Other drugs also can cause addiction, preterm birth, or mental problems. Protecting your baby is a great reason to quit! (See pages 29 through 33.)

Get enough folic acid every day

Folic acid helps prevent very serious brain defects and spina bifida.* Every woman who could get pregnant should get at least .4 milligrams (400 mcg) of folic acid every day.

You can get folic acid (also called folate) from many foods. Some examples are dark green leafy vegetables, broccoli, orange juice, some dry cereals, kidney beans, and liver. It is hard to get enough from foods. That is why **it is important to take a vitamin pill every day before you get pregnant.** Ask your health care provider which kind of vitamin pill is best.

If you have had a baby with spina bifida or anencephaly (no brain), talk with your health care provider. You probably should take even more folic acid before you get pregnant again.

*Spinal cord: The main nerve that carries messages about feeling and movement between your brain and body. It goes down your back inside the spine.

*Preterm birth: Early birth, before 37 weeks. The infant usually is small and has to stay in the hospital after birth. Many babies born very early have other health problems.

*Spina bifida: a very serious defect of the spine. It often prevents a person from walking.

15

Keeping track of your periods

It is a good idea to keep a record of your menstrual periods* before you get pregnant. Know the date each period began and how long each cycle* lasted. This helps you know when your next period is late. It will also help you figure out when you will give birth.

Write in the date when your period starts each month on the chart below—or on a calendar. Also count and write in the number of days of your cycle. This will help you know when to expect your next period.

*Menstrual period: The bloody flow from a woman's vagina that comes every month. Often called a "period."

*Cycle: The number of days between the start of one menstrual period and the start of the next. It is usually between 25 and 32 days long.

Menstrual Period Chart

1. Date period started _____
   Month, date

2. Next period started _____
   Month, date

   Length of your cycle (number of days since your last period started) _____

3. Next period started _____
   Month, date

   Length of your cycle _____

4. Next period started _____
   Month, date

   Length of your cycle _____

5. Next period started _____
   Month, date

   Length of your cycle _____

How do I know if I'm pregnant?

Some of the first signs of pregnancy:

- missed menstrual period
- tiredness
- tender, swollen breasts
- upset stomach

If you have two or three of these signs, you might be pregnant. Get a pregnancy test if your period is at least two weeks late. **During these early weeks, take care of yourself as if you were pregnant.** This is the first step toward being healthy while you are pregnant.

If you have a positive pregnancy test, it is time to get a physical exam. Make an appointment with your doctor, nurse-midwife, or clinic right away.

How do I get a pregnancy test?

You can buy a home pregnancy test kit at a drug store or go to your doctor or clinic for a test. Some clinics, like Planned Parenthood, may offer free pregnancy tests.

The home test can be done soon after your menstrual period is late.

If a home test shows that you are **not** pregnant, wait a week or two. If your period does not come, get a second test. Then see your provider to find out why your period is late. If you are not pregnant, this could be a sign of other health problems.

Now that I'm pregnant, what next?

This is a time when you may feel both excited and scared. Most women have mixed feelings—and many questions.

How will a baby change my life?

Will my baby be healthy?

What will birth be like?

Will I know how to be a good parent?

You will not learn the answers to all these questions right away. **What you can do now is begin to live in a healthy way.**

Look ahead to Chapters 2, 3, and 4. They will help you get started. Chapter 4 tells you more about the first few months of pregnancy. Look on page 10 for a keepsake page. Here you can write down special memories of this time. In the Purple Pages at the back, you will find ideas about places to get help in your community and a list of other books to read.

Every baby is special!

If this will be your first baby, you are starting a new adventure—parenthood. If you have other children you know that every baby is one-of-a-kind and every pregnancy is different.

You might have twins or even more than two babies. This is happening more and more today. In this book we will talk mostly about a single baby, because most women still have one baby at a time.

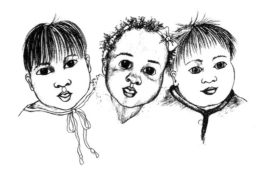

What is happening to me?

Your body is starting to change in many ways. Your belly may not start to grow bigger for another month or two. But you will probably begin to feel different right away. These signs are normal:

- Your menstrual periods have stopped. You are already about 2 weeks pregnant when you miss your first period!
- Your breasts may swell and become tender.
- You may feel more tired than usual.
- You may need to urinate more often than before.
- Your stomach may feel upset or you may vomit your food.
- You may lose a little weight.
- Your moods may change quickly. You may feel like crying one minute and be very happy the next.

How do you feel about having a baby?

✔ *Check all that you feel, or write in your thoughts:*

_____ It's wonderful.

_____ It feels strange.

_____ I can't quite believe it.

_____ I don't feel ready to have a baby.

I am a little bit afraid of _____

_____

_____

I am worried about _____

_____

_____

When will my baby be born?

A baby takes about 40 weeks to grow after the date of your last period. Your "due date" is when your baby is likely to be born. Here is how to find your due date.

Write down the date your last menstrual period started.

1. Date of your period   _____ _____

                                   Month   *day*

2. Add 7 days: + 7 days

3. Add 9 months: + 9 months

4. Your baby's due date: _____ _____

                                   Month   *day*

You may not know exactly when your last period started. Your doctor or nurse-midwife can tell about when your baby is due by:

- the size of your uterus,*
- the results of an ultrasound* test,
- the date when your baby's heartbeat is heard for the first time,
- the date when you first feel him move.

*Uterus:
The part of a woman's body where the unborn baby grows.

*Ultrasound:
A method of seeing inside the uterus or other part of the body. This test uses sound waves that make a picture on a TV screen.

Your baby could come early—or late

Most babies come some time between 2 weeks before and 2 weeks after their due dates. Be ready a few weeks before the date, in case your baby comes early.

Only your body knows for sure when your baby will arrive! You will have some signs, but even your doctor or nurse-midwife can't tell for sure.

If you are a single woman...

You do not have to go through this time by yourself. **Good friends and family members can be wonderful support during pregnancy and birth.** Find one or two people who will listen to your feelings. Take time to choose a birth partner who will be with you when your baby is born.

If you are a teenager...

At this time you will be facing big changes in your life. You will have to make serious choices and new plans. You may find it hard to know what is best.

Getting a pregnancy test early and starting prenatal care right away is important. You will need to find out where to go for health care. You may want to talk with someone you trust about your feelings. You could talk with:

- your parents,
- a nurse or advisor at school,
- your regular doctor, nurse, or community clinic,
- a person you trust at your place of worship.

If you are not sure you are ready to be a parent...

Talk with a professional you trust about the choices you have. Whatever you choose, be sure to take good care of your health now.

To fathers:
This is your pregnancy, too!

Share these pages with your baby's father. Encourage him to read the whole book as your pregnancy goes on. There are other pages with special notes for fathers, too.

As a father-to-be, you have a special part to play. Your wife or partner and your unborn child both need your help.

The most important thing you can do is to give mother and baby your loving support. One way you can help is to learn about pregnancy. Another is to help her practice healthy habits.

You may not have learned much about being a father from your own dad. Learning more will help you overcome many fears. Start with this book. It will give you the facts about pregnancy, delivery, and caring for a new baby.

After the birth, you can do as much for your baby as mom can—except for breastfeeding. Take your turn with the ordinary tasks of parenting. Cuddling, burping, and changing diapers will help you and your baby feel close. From the start, you are a very important part of your child's world.

Fathers-to-be often wonder:

- Am I being left out of the excitement?
- Do my partner's moods mean she's angry with me?
- Will we still enjoy sex as pregnancy goes on—and afterward?
- Will I be able to stay in the delivery room without fainting?
- Will I be a good father?

If something worries you, tell your partner about it. Talking together may help answer some of your questions. It is important for each of you to know what the other is thinking.

You also may want to talk with the doctor or nurse-midwife. Friends who are already parents can share what they have learned.

How can a father take part?

Here are some things you can do in the first months of your baby's life.

- **Learn as much as you can about pregnancy and being a parent.**
- Encourage your baby's mother to eat healthy foods. Try to eat well yourself.
- **Help her avoid smoking, drinking alcohol, or taking any other drugs.** Find other things to do together. Plan visits with friends, listen to relaxing music, or take her for a picnic.
- Go with your partner to prenatal checkups.
- **Go to childbirth classes** with her. You will learn what to expect and how to help during birth.
- Take walks and do prenatal exercises with her.
- Share home chores, like laundry, cooking, and cleaning.
- Avoid joking or criticizing your partner's changing body shape. Many women worry about how their bodies look. Her weight gain is for her baby's health.
- **Talk over your feelings about becoming parents.** Let her know about your excitement and concerns. Listen to her feelings. Give her an extra hug if she is feeling unhappy.
- In the later months, put your hand on her belly. You will feel your growing baby move inside.
- **Talk to your baby.** Unborn babies can hear voices during the last months before birth. Your baby will learn to know your voice.

■ ■ ■ ■ ■ ■ ■ ■ ■ ■

Tip–Smoke can harm unborn babies:

If you smoke, do it outside, away from your baby's mother. This would be a great time for you to quit!

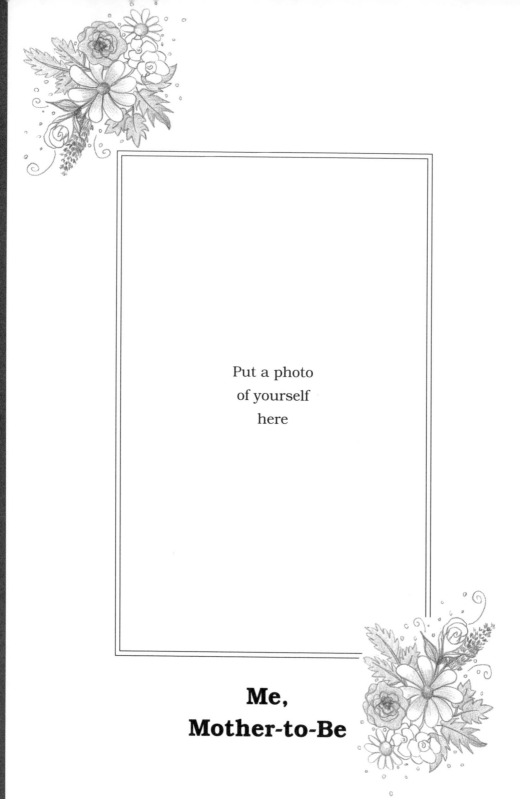

Put a photo
of yourself
here

Me,
Mother-to-Be

Chapter 2

Staying Healthy

Here are the most important things you can do to keep yourself and your unborn child healthy.

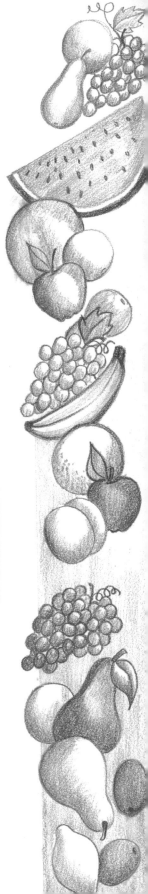

Healthy Habits

1. Go to all your health checkups.

2. Don't use alcohol, cigarettes, or drugs.

3. Eat healthy foods.

4. Protect yourself from disease during sex.

5. Buckle your safety belt every time you ride in a car, truck, or van.

6. Exercise regularly.

7. Learn to relax and accept all your feelings.

These healthy habits apply to anyone, woman or man, young or old. If you can follow them while you are pregnant, you will be healthier throughout life.

You will find more in this chapter about how these things affect your baby. The way he or she grows and changes is called "development."

If I'm feeling fine, why do I need prenatal checkups?

"Prenatal care" is health care during pregnancy. At prenatal checkups, your doctor or nurse-midwife will see how you and your baby are changing. She will look for health problems that you may not be able to feel.

If your health is good, you will have one checkup each month. In the last two months before birth, you will be checked more often.

Your health care provider will check:

• the baby's growth, heart rate, and movement;

• how you feel and how your body is changing;

• your weight gain and food habits;

*Blood pressure:
The force of the blood pumped by the heart through your blood vessels. High blood pressure means the heart is working extra hard.

• your blood pressure* and urine for signs of health problems; other tests will be done, too;

• any minor problems that make you feel ill or uncomfortable.

The chances are good that you will have no serious problems. **But a serious problem is easiest to treat if it is found early.** Your provider will take special care before, during, and after birth to lessen any problems.

Preterm birth is one of the most important things to prevent. A baby who is born too early can have many serious health problems. There are things you can do to reduce your chance of preterm birth, like eating nutritious foods and not smoking. Your provider will do all she can to help you. Learn the warning signs for preterm labor. (See page 86.)

Your doctor or nurse-midwife wants to hear from you. **The checkup is your best time to ask questions.** As you go through this book, you will find places to write down questions you want to ask. Ask any questions that you think of. This is no time to be shy! For more information about checkups and finding a provider, see Chapter 3.

Introducing your unborn baby

Here are life-sized pictures showing the growth of an unborn baby in the first four months. See how quickly a baby grows! All the main parts of the body are formed very early. This is why you need to take care of yourself during this time.

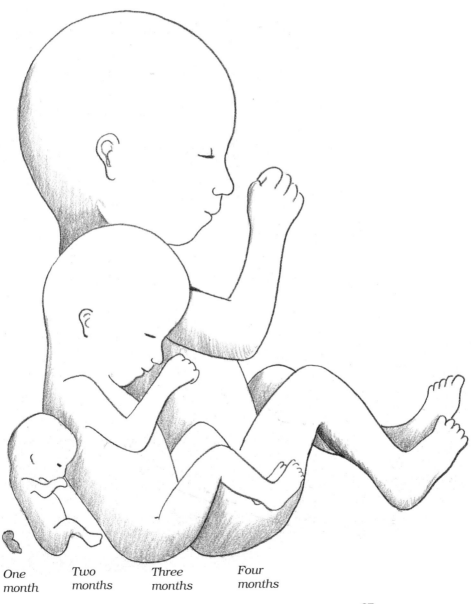

One month   *Two months*   *Three months*   *Four months*

How healthy are my habits?

Most of us have some habits that help an unborn baby. Some of our other habits could be unhealthy. Mark the boxes of the list of healthy habits below. Be honest with yourself—for the health of your baby!

Yes	No	Healthy Habits
❏	❏	I eat 5 or more servings of fruits and vegetables daily.
❏	❏	I drink at least 8 glasses of water and other liquids every day.
❏	❏	I have stopped smoking.
❏	❏	I do not drink beer, wine, wine coolers, or hard liquor.
❏	❏	I take no drugs, except those my doctor has prescribed.
❏	❏	I get about 7 to 8 hours of sleep every night.
❏	❏	I exercise for about 30 minutes at least 3 times a week.
❏	❏	I take some time to relax every day.
❏	❏	I talk over my worries with others.

Did you answer "no" to any questions above? Those are the most important things for you to try to change while you are pregnant. Write down the habits you want to change:

_____

_____

_____

Nobody's perfect, but you are making a good start!

You may need help in making these changes. **Talk with your doctor, nurse, nurse-midwife, or another person you trust.**

Medicines and other drugs can cause harm

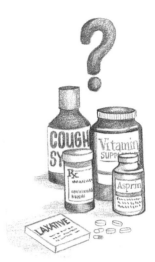

Your baby can be affected by almost anything you eat, drink, or breathe. Healthy food and fresh air are the substances your baby needs and gets through your body.

Many other things you take into your body are drugs.* How often do you take an aspirin pill or a spoonful of cough medicine? When was the last time you had a cup of coffee or sat in a smoky room?

If you are pregnant, any of these could harm your baby. Remember that your unborn child is much smaller than you. Even a very small amount of some drugs could do harm.

Check with your doctor or nurse-midwife before taking any medicines, including:

- pills or other medicines prescribed by a doctor,
- aspirin, vitamin pills, laxatives, and other medicines you can buy without a prescription.

Breaking habits

Some drugs, especially alcohol, tobacco, and most illegal drugs, could cause very serious health effects both to you and your baby. Many of those things are also habit-forming. **If you have a habit you can't break by yourself, now is the time to get help.**

It is important for your health care provider to know about any drugs you may use. Try to be honest with her. She will know where you can get treatment.

*Drugs: Chemicals that change the way your body feels or works. These include alcoholic drinks, cigarettes, coffee and other caffeine drinks, prescription and over-the-counter drugs, as well as illegal drugs.

How does alcohol harm babies?

Of course no mother would try to harm her unborn baby. However, if you drink beer, wine, or mixed drinks, the alcohol goes from your blood stream into your baby's body. If you get high or drunk, your unborn child will, too.

Alcohol can hurt the brain before birth. It can slow the unborn baby's growth and give him other problems. Children who have been harmed by alcohol before birth can have problems with health, learning, and behavior. This is called Fetal Alcohol Syndrome.*

*Fetal Alcohol Syndrome: The severe health and developmental problems of a child who has been damaged by alcohol before birth. It includes both mental retardation and physical defects. Also called "FAS."

Serious harm can be done when the baby is just starting to grow inside. **It is important to stop drinking as soon as you think you might be pregnant.** Alcohol can affect your baby's development all through pregnancy. It can harm a baby who is breastfeeding, too.

No one knows how much a woman can drink safely, so it is best not to drink at all. Even a little alcohol may harm a baby to some degree. You don't have to be an alcoholic to have a child affected by alcohol.

Did you know?

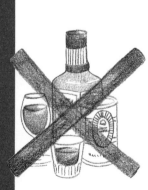

- A woman's blood absorbs more alcohol from a drink than a man's does. The same size drink will affect you more than a man.

- **There is the same amount of alcohol in a can of beer, a bottle of wine cooler, a glass of wine, and a shot of hard liquor.**

- "Coolers" and many mixed drinks may taste like soft drinks. They often have a lot of alcohol in them, however.

- Fetal Alcohol Syndrome is the most preventable kind of mental retardation.

Is it hard to quit drinking?

If you are not able to stop drinking easily, you may need help. Talk with your family about your effort to stop. Your doctor or nurse-midwife can help you get counseling. **It may be hard to quit, but it will be best for both you and your baby.**

Tips to make quitting easier:

• Stay out of places where people are drinking.

• If others in your family drink, let them know why you are trying not to drink. Ask them to do other things with you. You could get some exercise or cook a nice dinner together.

• If you feel like drinking when you are alone, find something else to do. Go see a friend who does not drink, take a walk, or see a movie.

This important time in your life is also the best time to quit drinking!

Drinking and driving can hurt, too!

Both you and your baby could be hurt if you drink and drive. Riding with someone who has been drinking is also risky. If you are injured, your unborn baby could easily be harmed.

If your driver has been drinking, you and your baby will be safer if you:

• Drive yourself.

• Take a cab home.

• Ask for a ride with someone who has not been drinking.

• Stay where you are.

• **Be sure to buckle your seat belt on every ride.**

How do cigarettes affect babies?

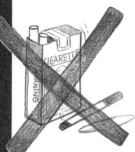

Your baby needs the oxygen in clean air. This oxygen is passed to his body by your blood. Every time you puff on a cigarette, carbon monoxide* and nicotine get into your blood. The blood carries those substances to your unborn baby. Nicotine makes his heart beat faster. Carbon monoxide takes the place of oxygen in his blood.

Babies of smokers often are smaller than other babies because they get less oxygen. After birth, they also may have problems. They may have more colds, lung illness, and ear aches than other children. Some may learn more slowly in school.

Your smoking could also cause a miscarriage* or make your baby be born early.

*Carbon Monoxide: A poisonous gas that results from burning tobacco or other things.

*Miscarriage: The loss of a baby born too early to survive outside the uterus. Most miscarriages happen less than 10 weeks after a pregnancy begins.

Other people's smoke

Breathing smoke from someone else's cigarettes affects your health. **It also reaches your baby's body and can cause harm**. If your friends smoke, ask them not to smoke in your home. And stay out of smoky places.

Caffeine in coffee, tea, and colas

Coffee, tea, and cola drinks have caffeine in them. **When coffee makes you feel jumpy, your baby gets that way, too.** More than one cup of coffee per day may help cause miscarriage. Caffeine also limits the vitamins and minerals a woman gets from food. If you like these drinks, use only a little.

A large amount of caffeine is found in many cold medicines, diet pills, and headache pills. It is also put in soft drinks like Coca Cola, Pepsi, Mountain Dew, and Dr. Pepper.

Illegal drugs and babies

Illegal drugs, like cocaine, heroin, PCP, and others, can be very dangerous for unborn babies. When a pregnant woman gets high, her unborn baby does, too. **What might make you feel good for a short time may do life-long harm to your child.**

Using these drugs even a few times could harm an unborn child. **If you have a drug habit, now is the time to get help and quit.** It may not be easy, but having a healthy baby is worth it!

Cocaine and crack—What they can do

Cocaine or crack use by a pregnant woman can cause:

- an early miscarriage
- heavy bleeding late in pregnancy
- preterm birth* and serious problems after birth
- a baby to be born addicted and go through the pain of withdrawal
- a child who has trouble learning or behaving as other children do

*Preterm birth: Early birth, before the unborn child is 37 weeks old. Preterm babies are more likely to have health problems than babies born after 37 weeks. Another word for preterm is "premature."

Marijuana

Smoking marijuana may cause preterm birth and the problems that go with it. There may be other unknown dangers. Other drugs are often added to marijuana before it is sold.

The sooner you stop smoking, drinking, or taking any drugs, the better for both of you.

Smart eating for baby and you

Nutritious foods help your body stay strong and your baby's body and brain develop well.

Eating well takes some planning. You may have to change some of your habits. To find foods you like that are also healthy for you:

- Think about the foods you eat now. Are they nutritious? Eat more of the healthy foods and less of the others.
- Try a new food each week.
- Before you go to the grocery store, make a list of healthy foods you want to eat. Make sure to buy at least some of them on each shopping trip.
- Eat some foods that are not your favorites. Do this for your baby. You may grow to like them.

*Organs: Parts of the body, including the heart, brain, stomach, uterus, liver.

*Cells: The billions of tiny things that make up all the parts of your body. There are many kinds of cells. Each does a special job to make your body work.

Seven nutrients your body needs

1. **Protein**—for growth of muscles, organs,* and cells.*
2. **Carbohydrates**—for energy.
3. **Fat**—for energy and cell growth.
4. **Vitamins**—for making the organs, muscles, nerves, and other parts of your body work right.
5. **Minerals**—for healthy growth of cells in bones, teeth, and blood.
6. **Fiber**—for better digestion of foods and prevention of certain diseases.
7. **Water**—for normal working of the entire body. All body cells contain a lot of water.

Certain foods have large amounts of these nutrients. They are the best ones to have every day. What are they? See the next page.

The healthy foods

Here are the kinds of foods that give you the most nutrients. It is best to eat a wide variety of foods. See the number of daily servings listed.

How many of these do you eat now?

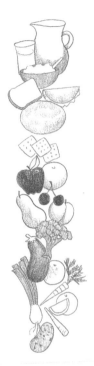

- **Breads and grains** (6 servings or more daily)

  Wheat bread, corn tortillas, rice, pasta, rye crackers, noodles, and cooked or dry cereal. Eat whole grains like brown rice and whole wheat bread every day. They have more nutrients than white bread, white rice, or spaghetti.

- **Fruits** (2 to 4 servings) **and vegetables** (3 to 5)

  Oranges, papaya, melons, prunes, broccoli, squash, potatoes, tomatoes, spinach, collard greens, and bok choy. Bright yellow, orange, or dark green vegetables and fruits are best. Fresh or frozen ones are better than canned.

- **Milk foods** (3 to 4 servings for pregnant women)

  Milk, hard cheese, cottage cheese, and yogurt. Non-fat or low-fat milk is better than whole milk. If milk makes you feel ill, see page 38 for other calcium foods.

- **Meats and beans** (2 to 3 servings)

  Fish, chicken, pork, eggs, lentils, peanuts, garbanzo beans, black-eyed peas, and tofu.

- **Water and other liquids** (8 tall glasses)

  Water is best. You can include milk and a little juice and thin soup. Coffee, tea, and regular or diet sodas don't count.

These foods are the best for everyone to eat.
But many people do not have enough water, grains, fruits, and vegetables in their diets. Most have too much fat and sugar.

What foods should I eat every day?

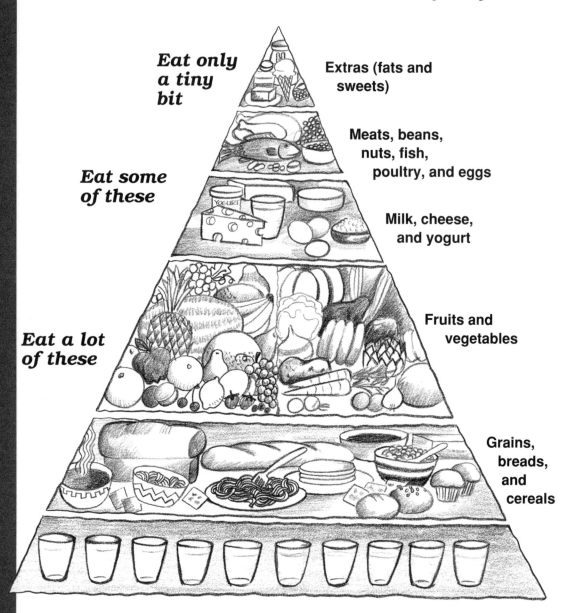

Eat only a tiny bit — Extras (fats and sweets)

— Meats, beans, nuts, fish, poultry, and eggs

Eat some of these — Milk, cheese, and yogurt

Eat a lot of these — Fruits and vegetables

— Grains, breads, and cereals

The Food Pyramid

The foods at the base are the most important part of a healthy diet. Eat plenty of them. Eat less of the foods near the top. The "extras" at the very top give you few nutrients. Eat as little of them as possible.

How big is a serving?

A small bowl of food for one person may seem like a huge meal to another. Try measuring foods to see how big a serving is. Read the labels on packages, too. Some examples are:

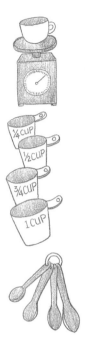

Fruit: 1 medium orange, ½ cup applesauce, ¾ cup juice

Vegetables: 1 cup raw lettuce, ½ cup cooked squash, ¾ cup juice

Grains: 1 slice of bread, ½ cup rice, 1 ounce (½ to 1 cup) dry cereal

Meats and beans: 2 to 3 ounces meat, poultry or fish (the size of a pack of cards), two eggs, 1 cup cooked kidney beans or lentils

Milk foods: 1 cup milk or yogurt, 1½ ounces (a slice) cheddar cheese, 2 cups cottage cheese

Extras: 1 tablespoon margarine, catsup, jelly, or salad dressing

Eating many kinds of foods

Eat many different foods during the day and from day to day. Eating the same things every day will not give you enough of the nutrients you need.

Often one dish will give you one serving of several types of food. For instance:

- spaghetti with tomato and meat sauce topped with grated cheese

- a bean burrito, with a flour tortilla, refried beans, cheese, lettuce, tomato, and salsa

- a stir-fry dish of chicken, broccoli, onions, bok choy, and carrots served with brown rice

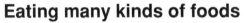

Tip–WIC: The **Women, Infants, and Children Program,** called "WIC," is an excellent service. Many pregnant women use it for nutritious foods and prenatal and infant care information. Call your local health department for more information.

Eat plenty of calcium

While you are pregnant, you need to eat plenty of calcium. Calcium makes your baby's bones and teeth strong. It also keeps your bones strong.

Milk has more calcium than most foods. But many adults find that milk gives them gas, cramps, and diarrhea.* This is called "lactose intolerance." It is very common among African-American, Hispanic, Asian-American, and Native-American people. **Tell your doctor or nurse-midwife if milk makes you feel sick.**

*Diarrhea: Bowel movements that come more often than normal. May be very soft and watery.

If you have lactose intolerance, you may be able to digest* some foods made from milk. Try yogurt with live cultures, or hard cheese like cheddar or Swiss. You may find "low lactose" milk and milk custard or pudding easier to eat. Your health care provider may suggest lactaid or calcium pills.

*Digest: To change the food you eat into substances your body can use. This is done in your mouth, stomach, and intestines.

These foods also give you plenty of calcium:

✔ collard greens, kale, cabbage, radishes, bok choy, parsnips, and broccoli; also orange juice with calcium added

✔ canned salmon or sardines with bones

✔ tofu made with "calcium sulfate" (see the label)

✔ corn tortillas made with lime; cooked dry beans

✔ blackstrap molasses; sesame seeds and peanuts

Folic acid—Be sure you get enough!

Folic acid (folate) helps your unborn baby be healthy. (See page 15.) Each day during pregnancy you should have at least .4 milligrams (or 400 mcg). This is the amount in most prenatal vitamin pills. You can get some from foods like dark leafy vegetables, orange juice, and dry cereals. It is hard to eat enough, so taking a vitamin pill every day is best.

Other food tips

- **If you are under age 18, you need extra protein and foods with calcium,** like cheese and milk. This is because your own body is still growing. These foods build your bones and muscles as well as your baby's body.

- **Vitamin and mineral pills do not take the place of healthy foods.** Foods have many other important nutrients in them, like fiber. Your doctor or nurse-midwife may want you to take specific vitamins or minerals, like calcium or iron.

- **Too much of some vitamins** can lead to problems in your pregnancy. Vitamin A is one of these. Only take as many vitamin pills as your health care provider advises.

- **Raw or undercooked meat, poultry, fish, eggs, or shellfish (clams and oysters)** may have tiny organisms* in them. These could make you or your unborn baby very sick.

  Cook these foods completely to kill all the organisms. Also, wash your hands well after handling raw foods. Wash the cutting board, too.

  *Organisms: Bacteria, viruses, or parasites. These are killed by cooking.

- **Avoid eating too many salty foods.** You can salt your food to your taste, unless you have certain problems with your pregnancy. But some foods, like chips, pickles, and packaged foods have very large amounts of salt. Look on the label for the amount of "sodium." Even some things that do not taste salty contain it.

- **Eating things that are not foods, like dirt, clay, or laundry starch, can be harmful when you are pregnant.** This is called pica. Some women like to eat things that are not food when they are pregnant. If you feel like this, tell your doctor or nurse-midwife.

  These things do not give you the nutrition you need. If you eat them, your baby may not get enough of the foods she needs to develop well. Eating some of these things can give you other health problems.

39

Healthy foods for life

Now is a good time to cut down your use of fats. This would keep your whole family healthier throughout life.

Cutting down on fats helps keep your heart healthy. You can do this by:

- eating less fried food
- taking smaller servings of salad dressing
- putting less butter or margarine on your bread

Saturated fats are more likely to harm your heart than others. Foods that are low in these fats include:

- low-fat milk, yogurt, and cottage cheese—instead of milk products containing cream
- soft margarine—instead of butter
- liquid cooking oils, like olive, peanut, corn, and soybean oil—instead of lard or coconut oil
- fish, chicken, and turkey—instead of hamburger or steak

Eating out, eating wisely

Restaurant meals are often loaded with fats and lacking in the nutritious foods you and your baby need. If you eat out often, choose the places and the menu items that will be best for you. Look for:

- foods that are not too spicy or oily
- a salad bar
- salad dressing "on the side" so you can add as little as you want
- main dishes of fish or chicken, broiled or baked rather than fried or covered with thick sauces

Keeping sex safe

While you are pregnant, it is nice not to have to think about birth control. But it is still very important to protect yourself from any "sexually transmitted diseases" or STDs. **STDs are diseases that spread from one person to another during sex.** Herpes, chlamydia, syphilis, gonorrhea, hepatitis B, and AIDS are all STDs.

Any of these diseases could harm your unborn baby as well as you. They can cause many problems, from serious eye infections or birth defects to fatal illness.

There are cures for most STDs. **If you are treated, your partner must also be treated or you may get sick again.**

Your doctor or nurse-midwife will test you for some of these diseases at your first checkup. If you think that you may have an STD, be sure to tell your provider.

Since most STDs can be treated, your baby can be born healthy.

AIDS is the most serious STD because it has no cure at this time. Treatment can keep it from spreading from mother to unborn baby.

Preventing STDs

Not getting an STD is better for your health than curing one. Three ways to prevent STDs are:

1. Having only one faithful sex partner for many years.

2. Not having sex at all.

3. Using a condom and a spermicide,*every time you have sex. This is not as safe as the first two suggestions.

*Spermicide: A cream or jelly used with a condom to kill germs as well as sperm that could be passed during sex.

41

Buckling up for both of you

Car travel seems so safe, but driving to the grocery store or mall may be the most dangerous part of your day. It is the biggest danger you and your unborn child face.

Motor vehicle crashes are the most common cause of death and injury to young men and women. **If you are hurt in a car, van, or truck crash, your baby may be hurt, too.**

Safety belts will give both of you good protection if you wear them correctly.

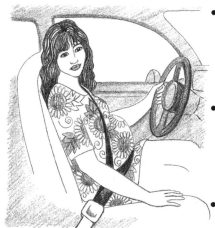

Buckling the lap and shoulder belts snugly keeps Mom and unborn baby protected.

- **Use both the lap and shoulder belts.** The shoulder belt greatly increases your safety. It keeps your head from being thrown against the windshield or dashboard.

- **Push the lap belt down under your belly, touching your thighs.** Pull it tight. The shoulder belt should be snug over your shoulder and across your chest. (See the picture.)

- **If your car has an air bag, it works with your safety belt** to protect your head and chest in front-end crashes. The air bag is a safety cushion built into the steering wheel or dashboard. In a front-end crash, it fills with air instantly. Your safety belt holds you in place during roll-overs and rear-end or side crashes.

The air bag works best if you sit as far away from the steering wheel or dashboard as possible. Slide your seat back. This gives plenty of room for the air bag to inflate.

■ ■ ■ ■ ■ ■ ■ ■ ■ ■

Tip–Baby's car seat: After your baby is born, he or she will need a special car safety seat. (More on page 91.)

Why should I exercise?

There are many reasons to exercise regularly. Some ways it can help you are:

✔ It relaxes your mind as well as your muscles. It can help you sleep better.

✔ Exercise helps you have regular bowel movements.

✔ It can prevent or lessen backaches.

✔ Exercise keeps your blood flowing well. This keeps your legs from swelling. It may help prevent varicose veins* and hemorrhoids.*

✔ It may lessen illness by strengthening your immune system.

How to exercise during pregnancy

• **Do it often, three or four times each week, for real benefits. (See pages 78 and 79.)**

• Be sure you tell your doctor or nurse-midwife what kind of exercise you are doing or want to start doing.

• You can usually continue the kind of exercise you were doing before your pregnancy—in moderation. High-impact aerobics and risky sports are not advised. If you have not been exercising, try easy things like swimming or walking.

• Try not to get overheated. Stop if you feel dizzy or faint. Exercise when the weather is cool.

• Drink plenty of water before and afterward.

• **Walking is one of the best exercises.** It is also one of the easiest and costs nothing. The only equipment you need is a pair of flat, cushioned sport shoes. Walk for about a half-hour each time. Start slowly, then walk fast enough to sweat a little bit.

*Varicose veins: Blue, bulging veins, often in the legs and groin.

*Hemorrhoids: Bulging veins in your anus, where bowel movements come out.

Both *varicose veins and hemorrhoids are caused by problems with blood flow. They may ache or itch and often start during pregnancy.*

Learning to relax and lessen stress

How you think and feel affects your body. Keeping your mind free of stress helps you stay healthy. It may even help you get better if you are sick. Enjoying the little things in life can make the hard parts easier.

Some things about being pregnant may not be pleasant. You may have aches and pains. Changing your habits, such as smoking cigarettes or drinking alcohol, may make you unhappy. Pregnancy may add extra stress to your family or job.

Some things may be both exciting and scary, like thinking about raising your child. Others can give you joy. Feeling your unborn baby kick you in the ribs can be a thrill!

Helping yourself be more content

This must begin in yourself. **Learn what helps you relax. This will help you find your own way to enjoy life and cope with difficulties.** Some things you could do for yourself are:

- Take a nap or spend some time alone.
- Rest your hand on your belly and feel your baby moving.
- Talk gently to your unborn child.
- Learn to knit or sew so you can make a baby blanket or quilt.
- Watch funny movies that make you laugh a lot.
- Take a long, warm shower.
- Exercise.

How can other people help me?

We all live with others—in small families or large ones, with school friends, work friends, and neighbors. **These people are your "support system." They can help in many ways, now and after your baby comes.**

Your husband or partner can share your joy and your worries. He can rub your feet if they ache. He can help you learn to eat new foods. You can share the fun of choosing your baby's name.

Your parents, brothers and sisters, other relatives, and friends also can give you support and comfort. They will want to help you in their own ways.

Be sure to tell your doctor or nurse-midwife about any problems in your life. Changes in your job, a move to a new town, or family problems can give you a lot of stress. This can affect your health.

Telling people what you need

You may know that all these people care. But they may not know what they can do to help you. **Try to tell them what you want,** like this:

- "Today I am very tired. Could you please care for my little boy, so I can take a nap?"

- "Let's watch a funny movie, not a sad one."

- "Please help with the laundry. My back aches."

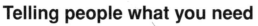

Tip–Both parents feel stress:

Remember, your baby's father may feel stress at this time, too. Give him extra hugs. You are in this together.

45

Trouble at home?
Help for abused women

Some women find that their husbands or partners hit, kick, or beat them. This dangerous abuse often begins or gets worse during pregnancy. Children in the family also might be attacked.

This is the crime called "domestic violence." It also is a serious health problem because it could harm both mother and unborn baby. The mother is not to blame. The person who attacks her is the one who is doing something wrong.

If this is happening to you, you do not need to take this abuse!

Getting help

- Call a crisis hotline. (Look up the number in the front of your telephone book, or call the local health department.)
- Tell a trusted friend, doctor or nurse, clergy member, or mental health counselor.
- **Find out where to get help in the community, such as a legal aid program or a counselor.**
- Learn about safe places to go if you need to leave. A battered women's shelter would give you protection.

Being a good friend

Do you know another woman who fears her husband or partner? Tell her of your concern and support her in getting help. **Women often hide signs of abuse.** Some signs you might look for:

- unexpected injuries blamed on "accidents"
- becoming less friendly or staying home alone most of the time
- increased alcohol or drug use

Can these things harm my baby?

Cat litter boxes?

Yes, cat feces* may have parasites that could infect you and your unborn baby. You may not feel sick, but your baby could be damaged.

Any kitten or cat that goes outdoors could catch these parasites. **Ask someone else to clean the litter box while you are pregnant**. If you work in the garden where cat feces may be, wear gloves.

*Cat feces: Cats' bowel movements; the parasites may give you toxoplasmosis. This can cause defects in a baby's body.

Lead in the air you breathe and in the water you drink?

Yes, lead may cause miscarriage or great harm to unborn babies and children. Lead* can be found in household dust, air, and water. It also is found in factories where painting or soldering is done.

*Lead: A metal that can cause very serious brain damage in infants and children.

- Do you work with lead? Ask for another job while you are pregnant or breastfeeding.

- Paint in older buildings has lead in it. You might breathe paint dust or eat tiny chips of paint without knowing it. A pregnant woman and her children should move out while paint in a home is being scraped or sanded.

- Lead in the pipes of old houses may leach into the water. Avoid drinking the water that has been sitting in the pipes overnight. Run the water for a few minutes in the morning before using it. Hot water absorbs more lead than cold water. When cooking and making coffee or tea, start with cold water.

Hot tubs, saunas, and steam rooms?

Yes, the very hot water or air might harm your baby by raising your body temperature. It is best not to use them while you are pregnant.

Could my work affect my baby?

This depends on the kind of job you have and how well you are feeling. What you can do about it depends on the company you work for.

Some problems during pregnancy could be made worse by your work. Some jobs could cause health problems. Here are things to think about.

- **Do you have a desk job?** Are you able to get up and move around during the day? If so, you are not likely to have serious job-related health problems.

*Toxic chemicals: Strong substances that could be poisonous to your unborn baby.

- **Do you face dangers in your job?** Are there toxic chemicals* or lead in your area? Do you work around X-rays, like in a dentist's office? All these things could cause problems in pregnancy. Ask to work away from such dangers if you can.

- **Does your job give your body a lot of stress?** Do you have to sit or stand all day? Do you have shift changes that make it hard to get enough sleep? Do you have to lift and carry heavy things? Are you required to work extra-long hours? You could:

*Support stockings: Hose with strong stretch that reduce swelling of your legs and help prevent varicose veins.

✔ Wear flat shoes and support stockings.*

✔ Do exercises like the pelvic tilt (page 78) to strengthen your back.

✔ Ask for rest times to walk around or put your feet up.

✔ Ask to be given another task.

Talk to your doctor and your employer if you think your health could be in danger. Ask your company to give you another task while you are pregnant. If you are having health problems, you may be able to get a leave of absence or disability leave.

Chapter 3

Choices in Prenatal and Birth Care

It is important to have a checkup at least once a month while you are pregnant. **Even when you are feeling well, you should see a doctor or nurse-midwife regularly.** These vists will help prevent problems that you may not feel.

Every pregnant woman needs a heath care provider and a place to give birth. You may have many choices or very few. This depends on where you live and on your health insurance plan. Some plans give you many options. Most have a list of hospitals and providers that you can use.

In some areas, there are hospitals, birth centers in hospitals, and separate birth centers. In small towns, there may be less choice. In some places, home birth is an option for women who are having normal pregnancies. Some insurance plans cover home births.

If you are not sure where to go for care, here are some places to call:
- your insurance benefits office
- local public health department
- community clinic

In Canada, your family doctor or a nurse-midwife, will care for you. If health problems come up, he or she may send you to a specialist.

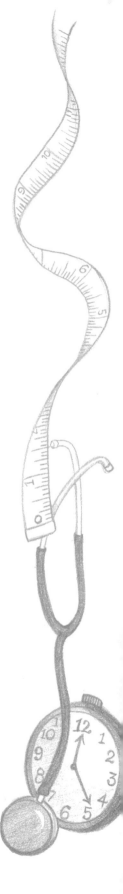

Where will my baby be born?

Some people start by choosing the place where they want to give birth. Others choose a health care provider first. **You need to know what services your health insurance covers.** Here are the basic differences between birth places.

Hospitals

Most babies are born in hospitals. **There you will get special care right away if problems come up.** Yet special care is not needed for most births.

Many hospitals:

- offer home-like birthing rooms
- allow your baby to stay in your room after birth
- allow birth partners to help you

Ask about these services before you choose a hospital.

Other options

Some parents want a more home-like kind of care. In some areas, delivery at a birth center or at home are simpler and lower in cost. **These choices are for women who expect to have a normal birth.** If a serious problem comes up during birth, the mother would be moved to a hospital right away.

Birth Centers: Some are in hospitals, others are separate. Nurse-midwives help women deliver their babies at birth centers. Find out which doctor and hospital would be used if problems develop.

Home: In a few places, some doctors and nurse-midwives will deliver babies at home. If you want to use a midwife, make sure she is certified. Also, make sure that the hospital to be used in an emergency is near your home.

Finding a doctor or nurse-midwife

Who will provide prenatal care* for you and help you deliver your baby? You will want to find a caregiver you like and trust. This person will help you through a very important time.

Find out if your health plan gives you a choice of providers. Ask for a list of those who are included.

The kinds of health care providers who give prenatal and birth care are:

Family physician: A doctor who gives primary (basic) care to people of all ages. Do you already have a doctor who takes care of your family? He or she may help you give birth and provide care for your baby.

Obstetrician-gynecologist: A doctor with special training in pregnancy, birth, and women's health. (Also called an "OB-GYN.")

Certified nurse-midwife: Providers specially trained as nurses and midwives. They are certified to provide prenatal and birth care. Many work in hospitals and in birth centers. Some do home births. (In some places, midwives who are not nurses are also certified to give care.)

You must ask questions to find a health care provider you like. Ask friends about the providers who helped deliver their babies. Would they use them again?

You may want to meet two or three providers before choosing. Ask them the questions on the next page. Look for a provider and staff who:

- are well trained and certified
- listen to your birth choices (see Chapter 7)
- have an office that is easy for you to get to
- have an office with easy access, if you have a disability

*Prenatal care: Regular checkups throughout pregnancy, as well as special care if health problems come up.

What to know before choosing a doctor or nurse-midwife:

There are some important things to know about your health care provider.

You will learn more if you know something about birth before asking these questions. This is a good time to read Chapter 7 and use the Glossary for help with medical words. Ask these key questions:

- ❏ Are you certified to help women to deliver babies?

- ❏ Do you have other doctors or nurse-midwives who care for your patients when you are away? Will I have a chance to meet them?

- ❏ Do you have a nurse I can call* days, nights, or weekends if I have a question or an emergency?

- ❏ Do you encourage women to deliver in the position that they find best for them?

- ❏ What methods do you prefer to use, if needed, to lessen pain during labor?

- ❏ How do you feel about a birth partner being with me for labor and delivery?

- ❏ Do you encourage a woman to try having a vaginal delivery if she has had a cesarean birth? (See page 123.)

If you are deaf or hard of hearing, you may want to know if "tty" access is available.

Do you have strong feelings about certain things, like episiotomy (page 121) or cesarean birth? Be sure to discuss them before choosing a provider.

Ask yourself: "Do I like this person and will I be able to trust him or her?" If you are not happy with your provider, talk with the customer service office of your health plan. Find out what options you have.

Talking with your provider

Remember that your health care provider wants to give you good care. But you must do your part, too. **Your part is to tell him* about things that worry you.**

*Him or her, or he and she, will be used to refer to a provider of either sex.

Write down concerns or questions as you think of them. (See the checkup pages in Chapters 4, 5, and 6.) This will help you remember to ask them at your next checkup.

Tell your doctor or nurse-midwife about changes you have noticed in your body. Tell her if you don't understand how to do what she has advised. Tell about the good things in your life and any problems you are facing.

If you feel sick...

Be sure to call your doctor or nurse-midwife. Note the answers to these questions before you call:

❏ How do you feel different from usual?

_____

❏ How long have you been feeling this way?

_____

❏ Have the feelings changed at all? _____

_____

❏ Do you have a fever? (Take your temperature and write it down before you call.) _____

Find mystery words in the Glossary

Health care providers may use medical words that you do not understand. Ask what they mean or look for them in the Glossary at the back of this book.

Your first prenatal checkup

Your doctor or nurse-midwife will give you a complete examination. She will:

- **Ask questions about your health habits.** Tell her as much as you can. Things you may not like to talk about could make a difference in your care. The same could be true for things that do not seem important to you. The more your provider knows, the better care she can give you.

- **Ask about the health of your parents** and relatives. Some health conditions found in your family could affect your health.

- **Check** your weight, temperature, heart rate, blood pressure, breasts, and lungs.

- **Give you a "pelvic exam."** This will show the size and health of your uterus and pelvis.

- **Get blood, urine, and other samples** to test for conditions like chlamydia, hepatitis B, and AIDS. Your provider needs to know about any problems as soon as possible.

An important test for HIV-AIDS

Many people who have HIV, the virus that causes AIDS, do not know it. A blood test for HIV is important for pregnant women because:

- A new treatment helps reduce the chance that an unborn baby will get HIV from his mother.

The pelvic exam is done while you lie on an exam table.

- If a woman has HIV, her provider can give her special care right away. Together they can plan the best care for her baby.

*Chronic disease: An illness that lasts a long time.

Your health care provider should talk with you about what the test means, before and after you take it. If you have HIV or AIDS, counseling can help you cope with this chronic disease.*

Chapter 4

Months 1, 2, and 3

Weeks 1 through 13

This chapter will help you through the first three months of your pregnancy. **Your whole pregnancy will last about nine months from your last menstrual period**. It is divided into three parts, called "trimesters." Chapters 4, 5, and 6 are about these trimesters, up through the eighth month. Chapter 7 covers the ninth month and birth.

Most women feel quite different during each trimester. The first is the time to get used to being pregnant. In the second, you settle down and feel quite content. In the third, you are looking ahead to birth and parenthood.

Doctors and nurse-midwives often talk about the weeks of pregnancy. This is because your baby grows and changes so much in each week of life. **There are about 40 weeks from your last period until birth.**

This is how the weeks and months add up:
1st trimester = months 1 - 3 = weeks 1 - 13
2nd trimester = months 4 - 6 = weeks 14 - 27
3rd trimester = months 7 - 9 = weeks 28 - 40

See how your body and your baby change

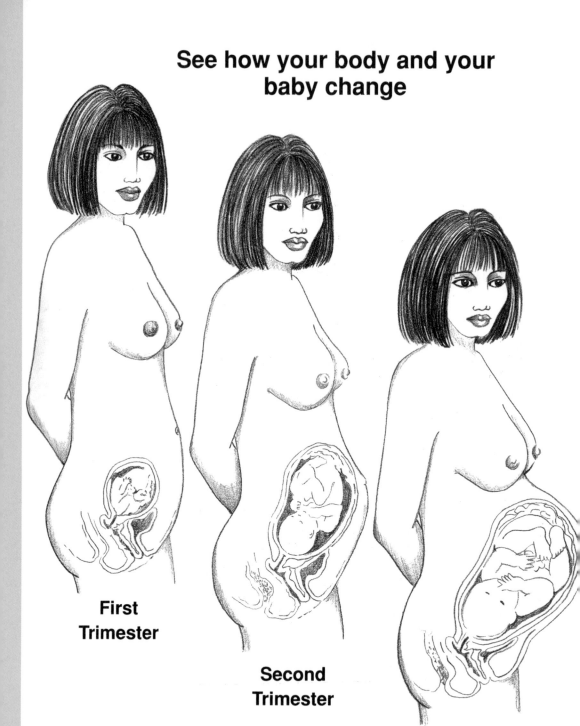

First Trimester

Second Trimester

Third Trimester

As your baby grows, your breasts swell and the top of your uterus pushes up higher in your body.

How is my baby growing?

Month 1 (1 to 5 weeks after your last period)

Your unborn baby (embryo) is too small to see at the beginning. In the first 4 weeks, he* grows to be almost as big as a peanut!

* Remember, this book will use "he" or "she" to refer to all babies, both male and female.

- His brain and spinal cord, lungs, and heart are forming.
- His head has little spots where his eyes will be.

Look back at the life-sized pictures on page 27. See the amazing growth now taking place.

Month 2 (6 to 9 weeks)

Now your unborn baby is beginning to look like a person. She has tiny eyes, ears, and a mouth. She grows to about one inch (25 millimeters) long, about the size of a walnut.

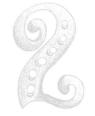

- She now has the beginnings of all the organs and systems that her body will have at birth.
- Legs and arms, tiny fingers, and toes are forming.
- Her brain is growing very fast so her head is much larger than her body.
- Her heart is beating, pumping blood in her body.

■ ■ ■ ■ ■ ■ ■ ■ ■ ■

Tip–Habits are hard to change: Now you know that smoking, drinking alcohol, or taking drugs can harm your baby. Are you finding it hard to quit using any of them? There are ways to break these powerful addictions.

Talk with your health care provider about ways to stop. Your health insurance plan or health provider probably offers programs to help people stop smoking. Your doctor or nurse-midwife also can help you get drug or alcohol abuse counseling.

My unborn baby's home

The organs of your body late in pregnancy. **Here is where your unborn baby grows!**

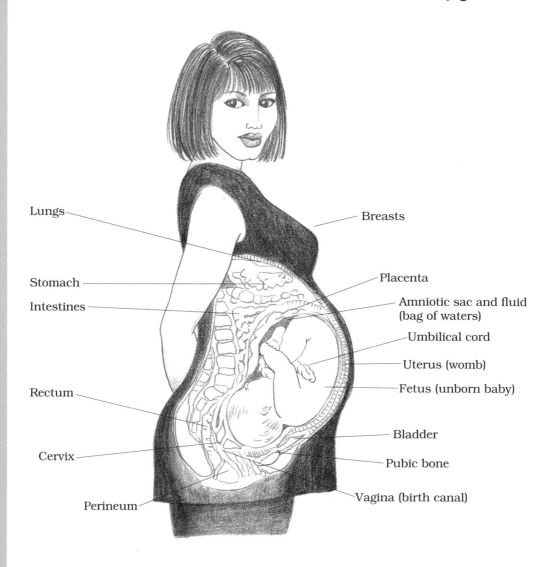

Lungs

Stomach

Intestines

Rectum

Cervix

Perineum

Breasts

Placenta

Amniotic sac and fluid (bag of waters)

Umbilical cord

Uterus (womb)

Fetus (unborn baby)

Bladder

Pubic bone

Vagina (birth canal)

The picture shows how, in the last three months, the growing baby will push against your lungs, stomach, intestines, rectum, and bladder. This can make you feel uncomfortable. (Read about these parts of your body on the next page.)

58

Your body and your baby

Your unborn baby lives in your **uterus** (womb). He is called an **embryo** during the first 8 weeks. After that, he is a **fetus**. He lies in the **amniotic sac** (bag of waters) filled with **amniotic fluid**.

The body parts in heavy black print on this page are shown in the drawing on page 58.

The **umbilical cord** and the **placenta** connect your baby's body to your body. The placenta is attached to the wall of your uterus. Food, oxygen, and other things your baby needs flow through the placenta and cord. Things that can harm your baby, like alcohol, also pass through the placenta into your baby's body.

At birth, the baby will be pushed down through the **cervix** (the opening of the uterus). He will be born through the **vagina** (birth canal). The birth canal passes between the pelvic bones (hip bones). The baby comes out through the **perineum** at the opening of the vagina.

Many organs are pushed out of place as your baby grows. These are normal ways your body will feel different when the baby gets larger:

- When your baby presses up against your **lungs**, you may feel short of breath.

- Your **stomach** and **intestines** may have a harder time digesting the food you eat. Large meals may make you uncomfortable.

- Your bowel movements may be harder to push out of your **rectum**.

- Your **bladder**, which holds urine, will be squeezed. You may need to urinate more often.

- Your **breasts** will swell and ache as they get ready to make milk after birth.

Your skin will also show some normal changes. Your skin may feel dry. A skin cream will help. Your face may break out or show changes in color across your nose and cheeks. You may get a dark line down the middle of your belly. Your nipples will get darker. Your breasts and belly may get stretch marks.

All about me

I am ___ years old. My birthday is _____.
(month, day, year)

I am _____ inches (___ centimeters) tall and
weighed _____ pounds (____ kilos) before I got
pregnant.

My last menstrual period started on _____.
(date)

- Health problems I have:

  _____

  _____

  _____

- Health problems in my family (husband or partner,
  my other children, my mother and father,
  brothers, sisters):

  _____

  _____

  _____

- **Questions I have about being pregnant**:

  _____

  _____

  _____

  _____

  _____

All of the things you have listed are important to
talk about with your doctor or nurse-midwife.

My first prenatal exam

On this date, _____ , I had my first examination (usually 4 to 8 weeks after your last period).

I am about ___ weeks pregnant.

I weigh ____ pounds (___ kilos) today.

My blood pressure is _____.

Tests I had today: _____

_____

_____

_____

My doctor or nurse-midwife's name* is

_____

Office phone:_____

Emergency phone:_____

*Put this name and both phone numbers in the front of this book and post them by your phone, so they will be easy to find.

Things I learned today

1. My baby's "due date" is _____

2. _____

_____

3. _____

_____

My next checkup will be on

the _____ of _____, at ____:____.
   (date)   *(month)*   *(time)*

■ ■ ■ ■ ■ ■ ■ ■ ■ ■

Tip–Saving your energy:
In the first few months, you may feel very tired. Learn to say "no" if you are asked to do something fun if you are feeling this way.

How can I take care of myself?

Some of your baby's most important growth happens in the first two months. Now is the time to remember and practice the healthy habits on page 25.

✔ Go to your checkups and learn about pregnancy.

✔ Don't smoke cigarettes, drink alcohol, or take drugs.

✔ Eat the healthy foods that your baby needs.

✔ Get plenty of exercise and rest.

✔ Make sure to protect yourself from STDs when having sex.

✔ Wear your safety belt on every car ride.

✔ Take time to relax.

What if my stomach feels upset?

In the early months, you may lose your appetite or feel like throwing up your food. This is called "morning sickness." It can happen at any time of day. It usually stops after the first few months. Here are some ways you can lessen it.

• Eat smaller meals and eat more often. Have something to eat before going to bed.

• Stay away from greasy or spicy foods.

• Eat plain crackers or fruit. Keep crackers beside your bed to eat before you get up.

• Sip a little plain soda water.

• Drink water or weak tea with a little sugar if you have been vomiting. This gives your body back the liquid it has lost.

• Always take your vitamins with food.

Call your provider between checkups if you are vomiting often!

Signs of an emergency...

Know how to reach your doctor or nurse-midwife. Call right away—day or night—if any of these things happen:

- **bleeding from your vagina**
- **painful cramps in your belly**
- **strong headaches, dizziness, vision problems**
- **fever or chills**
- **swelling of your hands, feet, or face**
- **very rapid weight gain**

Could I lose my unborn baby?

Some pregnancies do not last. About one-quarter of all pregnancies end with a miscarriage in the first three months. **Most miscarriages cannot be stopped. They usually are the body's way to deal with a baby who was very sick or not growing normally.** They are not caused by things you normally do. Working hard or having sex does not make a miscarriage happen.

After a miscarriage, you may feel very sad for weeks or months. This is normal. You have lost your unborn child. Other people may not understand your sadness, but it is very real. You may want to talk with others who have had miscarriages.

After your uterus heals, you can almost always get pregnant again. Talk with your doctor or nurse-midwife about how soon to try again.

Could my baby be born with a birth defect?

*Birth defect:
A health problem that begins before birth or soon after. Also called a "congenital defect."

A small number of babies have birth defects.* Many expectant parents worry about this. Some defects are serious, but others are not.

Causes of birth defects

- **A health problem of the mother.** (Example: If a mother has German measles in early pregnancy, her baby may have hearing, heart, and eye problems.)

- **Something that gets into the mother's body** and harms the unborn baby. (Example: Alcohol can cause serious defects in the brain and body.)

- **A genetic defect** that is inherited or passed along in a family. (Example: Sickle-cell anemia is a genetic disease.)

- **Many defects have unknown causes.**

*Amniocentesis:
A test of the fluid inside the bag of waters, showing certain things about your baby's health.

Some defects show up in special tests that can be done during the third to fifth month of pregnancy. These tests include ultrasound, special blood tests, and amniocentesis.* If the tests show a possible problem, the pregnant woman would have other, more exact, tests.

Do you know any members of your family who have had a birth defect? If so, you may want to talk with a genetics counselor.*

*Genetics counselor:
A person who can help you understand birth defects that have happened in your family and how they might affect your baby.

Ask your health care provider or genetics counselor if any of these tests would be helpful to you. Learn about the tests so you can decide if you want them. If your unborn baby has a defect that can be found, it is often helpful to know early. You and your health care providers can prepare to take the best care of your baby.

Check your health insurance policy or benefits office to find out what genetic services are covered.

Why do I feel happy one minute and sad the next?

In the first three months, you are likely to have strong feelings of sadness and happiness. This may surprise you. **This is normal and is caused by changes in the hormones* inside your body.** Most women's moods settle down after the first trimester.

*Hormones: Substances made by organs in the body that control how your body works and feels. During pregnancy there are major changes in hormones.

Things to do to help you feel better:

✔ Eat healthy foods.

✔ Get lots of exercise and rest.

✔ Talk about your feelings. This helps you, your family, and your friends understand these moods.

You may have fears or worries about your baby's health. These thoughts are normal, too. **Learning often makes you less afraid.**

- Are you worried about your baby's health? Learn more about the real risks and what you can do about many of them.

- Are you worried about what birth will be like? A childbirth class will help answer your questions. You can also read books and pamphlets. (See the list in the Purple Pages at the back of this book.)

- Are you worried about being a good parent? Start learning now about how to care for your baby. You may be able to practice by caring for a friend's baby.

■ ■ ■ ■ ■ ■ ■ ■ ■ ■ ■

Tip–Finding out more: You can find information about birth and infant care in many places. Look in the Purple Pages, page 152. Ask for a list of resources at your clinic. Stop in at your local library. The health department or WIC office can help. Community colleges often have classes for expectant parents. Look in the community pages in the front of your phone book.

Talking can help

Telling someone who cares about you often helps you feel better! This might be your baby's father, your mother, your sister, or your best friend. **Pick people who will really listen to you. They are more helpful than people who try to tell you what to do.** What two people would you want to tell most things?

1. _____

2. _____

How do you feel now?

_____

_____

_____

_____

What worries do you have?

_____

_____

What makes you feel happy now?

_____

_____

_____

Should I tell my doctor or nurse-midwife?

Yes, these people want to know about your moods and worries. Be sure to call if you feel like this for more than two weeks:

- You feel very sad or empty.
- You are not able to sleep or are sleeping all day long.
- You have no appetite or are eating all the time.

My third month (10 to 13 weeks)

How is my body changing?

- You are starting to gain some weight. By the end of this month, you probably will have gained 2 to 5 pounds (900 to 2200 grams) in all. You will need some larger clothes soon.

- By the end of this month, you may be able to feel your uterus. Press your fingers into your belly just above your pubic bone. You will feel something round and hard like an orange. That is the top of your uterus.

- Your breasts will probably feel very heavy and may hurt. This is normal. A bra that fits will help.

- You may get constipated more often than before you got pregnant.

How is my baby growing?

- By the end of this month, your baby will be about 4 inches (10 centimeters) long.

- Your baby will weigh about one-half ounce (15 grams) and is called a **fetus*** instead of embryo.

- His heart is beating very fast. It is loud enough for your doctor or nurse-midwife to hear.

- Fingers and toes are completely formed.

- Arms and legs can move now. Your baby is still so small that you cannot feel the kicks.

***Fetus:** the word for a unborn baby after 8 weeks of age.

■ ■ ■ ■ ■ ■ ■ ■ ■ ■ ■

Tip–Things your baby will need:

Now is a good time to start thinking about getting clothes, a car seat, and other baby things. It takes time to get everything a baby needs. See the lists on pages 90 through 92 for ideas. If you are looking for bargains, beware of second-hand car seats and cribs. They may have serious safety problems.

What can I do to stay healthy?

✔ Eat plenty of vegetables, fruits, and whole grain breads.

✔ Drink plenty of water instead of sweet soft drinks and diet sodas. For a change, try fruit juice with fizzy soda water.

✔ To get some exercise, walk to the store or to a friend's house instead of driving.

✔ Stay out of smoky rooms. Remember, smoke that you breathe can harm your baby. Ask friends not to smoke inside your home.

✔ Don't use medicines you have around the house. First ask your health care provider if they are safe to take. There may be ways to treat some health problems, like colds, without taking medicine.

Questions to ask at my next checkup

• What can I do if I am constipated?

• Why do I feel so happy and then so sad?

• Am I gaining enough weight?

• How will I know if I am having twins?

• I am having trouble quitting smoking. What will make quitting easier?

Other questions I have:

1. _____

2. _____

Monthly checkups

Your checkups will probably be simple and short. Your weight, blood pressure, and uterus size will be measured. A urine sample will be taken. Your provider will check your baby's heart beat. Soon you will be able to hear it, too. At some visits, you may have other tests, like ultrasound, to see how the baby is growing. You will have time to ask questions, too.

My three-month checkup

On this date, _____, I had my three-month appointment.

I am ___ weeks pregnant.

I weigh ___ pounds (___ kilos) now.

I have gained ___ pounds (___ kilos) since my last checkup.

My blood pressure is _____.

Things I learned today

1. _____

   _____

2. _____

   _____

3. _____

My next checkup will be on

the _____ of _____, at ___:___.
     (date)   *(month)*   *(time)*

■ ■ ■ ■ ■ ■ ■ ■ ■ ■

Tip–Having twins? Tests can be done to check this early in pregnancy. If you are having a "multiple" pregnancy, there are some extra risks. But with good care and healthy habits, you are very likely to have healthy babies.

You can expect to:

- gain more weight and be less comfortable
- need more rest – lying on your left side is best
- go to checkups more often later in pregnancy
- need to eat more nutritious foods
- be more likely to start labor too soon. (See preterm labor, page 86.)

Do I have to "eat for two"?

You do not need to eat twice as much as before you got pregnant. You **do** need to eat what your baby needs.

Most pregnant women need to eat only a little more than usual. The important thing is to eat healthy foods so you and your unborn baby get the best nutrition possible.

Will I gain too much weight?

It is healthy to gain weight while you are pregnant. You can see from the next page that many parts of your body get heavier as the months go by. Your body makes these changes to grow your baby and get ready for birth. Most women lose that weight after their babies are born.

It used to be considered healthy to gain as little weight as possible during pregnancy. Now we know that gaining too little weight can cause preterm birth. The baby may be born small for his age, which can cause health problems.

You can see that this is not the time to diet! If you limit the healthy foods you eat, your baby's food is limited, too. Also, diet pills are drugs that could be especially harmful to your unborn baby.

Are you afraid to gain weight? Do you diet a lot or make yourself vomit to stay thin? These habits could harm you and your baby's health. You can get help by talking about this problem with your doctor or nurse-midwife.

■ ■ ■ ■ ■ ■ ■ ■ ■ ■

Tip–Teens and weight gain: If you are a teenager, remember that your body is also still growing. You need to gain weight. Limit the junk food that is so easy to buy or fix. It may spoil your appetite for nutritious foods.

70

How much weight gain is healthy?

How much is best for you? That depends on your weight before you got pregnant. Your health care provider can answer that question best. A healthy gain for women of normal weight is between 24 and 34 pounds. If you are pregnant with twins, you can expect to gain more (40 to 60 pounds).

Gaining too little or too much could mean problems for your baby. You will be weighed at each checkup. Limit your food only if your doctor or nurse-midwife asks you to.

Your breasts have probably already gotten larger and heavier. Many other parts of your body will get heavier, too. The picture on page 58 shows these parts. The box below shows where all the weight goes.

Your Weight Gain During Pregnancy

Parts of the body	Weight at baby's birth
Your baby	7 to 8 pounds
Uterus - where your baby grows	2 pounds
Amniotic sac and fluid - surrounds your baby	2 pounds
Placenta - connects mother and baby	2 pounds
Breasts - ready to make milk	1 to 4 pounds
Extra blood in your body	4 to 5 pounds
Other fluids	3 to 5 pounds
Fat - stored energy for birth and breastfeeding	4 to 6 pounds
Total weight gain	**25 to 34 pounds**

Keeping up your healthy habits

Remember, even small changes will help give your baby a better start!

How are you doing now? You probably have been making some big changes in your life and activities.

Many pregnant women must work hard to change how they eat, sleep, or exercise. **It is hard to break old habits.** These might be eating too potato chips, smoking, drinking, taking drugs, or never getting any exercise. Have any of these things been hard for you?

What have been the hardest things to change?

_____

_____

What has been the easiest to change?

_____

_____

Who has helped you the most in making changes?

_____

_____

What healthy habits are you still working on?

_____

_____

_____

_____

■ ■ ■ ■ ■ ■ ■ ■ ■ ■

Tip–Would you like help? If you need help from your baby's father, your friends, and your family, ask for it. Many people will want to help you give your baby the best. They cannot always know what you need unless you tell them.

Chapter 5

Months 4, 5, and 6

Weeks 14 to 27

The second trimester of your pregnancy is beginning. Most women feel better and find these months to be easier than the first trimester. Your body is getting used to having a new life growing inside. You are getting used to the idea of being a mom.

This trimester is a time when your body will begin to change shape. Exercise becomes more and more important. By six months, you will be starting to plan for your labor and your baby's birth.

During this time, you can start thinking about caring for your baby after birth. You will need to decide whether you want to breastfeed your baby or use bottles. You will probably begin collecting the clothing and other things your baby will need.

As your body starts to change shape, your baby's father may become more interested in your pregnancy. **If you haven't done so already, share this book with him.** Invite him to come with you to your checkups.

Remember: Every prenatal checkup is important. If you miss a visit, call right away and set another date.

Getting ready for birth

Why start so early?

It is not too soon to begin getting ready for the big event—your baby's birth. **This is because it takes time to learn all you need to know. It also takes time for you to strengthen your birth muscles.**

Do you worry about what labor and delivery will be like? This is normal. You may have heard stories that scare you. Or you may have had a delivery that was hard. The best way to lessen fear is to learn about what is happening to your body. No birth is without pain and hard work, but the more you know, the less painful your labor will probably be.

How can I prepare myself?

The most important things you can do to get ready for birth are:

* **Birth partner:** A person who will be with you through labor and delivery. Having a trained birth partner, especially another mother, can help labor go well.

- **Choose a birth partner***—so you will have your baby's father or a close friend with you during labor. Having someone with you can be very comforting. This person must go to childbirth classes with you. You may be able to have more than one birth partner helping you.

- **Go to childbirth classes**—so you will know what labor and delivery are all about. Classes are given by hospitals, health clinics, and childbirth groups. Classes usually last six or eight weeks. You will need to sign up ahead of time. Take a class that meets at a time when your birth partner or partners can go with you.

- **Practice relaxation, exercises, and breathing**—so your body will be in the best possible shape.

My fourth month (14-18 weeks)

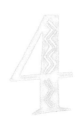

How is my body changing?

- You are starting to gain weight more quickly, and will gain about 1 pound each week from now on.
- Your breasts are still large, but may be less tender.
- You may not need to urinate as often as during the past months.
- If you had morning sickness, you may start to enjoy eating again.
- You may have more energy again.

How is my baby growing?

- At the end of this month, your unborn baby will be up to 7 inches long (18 centimeters). She will weigh about three-quarters of a pound (400 grams).
- Soft hair, called "lanugo," grows on her body. Eyebrows and eyelashes appear.
- She will be able to suck and swallow.
- You may start to feel some tiny kicks. They may feel like twitches or rumblings of gas.

■ ■ ■ ■ ■ ■ ■ ■ ■ ■

Tip–Delicious and healthy snacks:

- **Fresh fruits**—orange, banana, or papaya with non-fat yogurt on top
- **Dried fruits**—raisins, apricots, or prunes mixed with roasted pumpkin seeds, peanuts, or almonds
- **Raw vegetables**—carrots, tomatoes, or broccoli dipped in a little salad dressing
- **Popcorn**—with little or no margarine

What can I do to stay healthy?

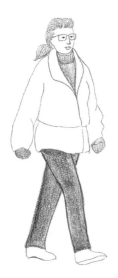

- Go for your regular checkups.
- Stay away from cigarettes, alcohol, or any drugs.
- Take a half-hour walk every day or two. For the best workout when you walk, go fast and swing your arms. Wear flat, cushioned sport shoes.
- Drink eight glasses of water every day.
- Have healthy foods on your kitchen shelf to have when you feel like a snack.
- Take only the vitamins or medicines that your doctor or nurse-midwife has told you to take. Take the right number each day. Remember, too much of some vitamins, like vitamin A, could be unhealthy for your pregnancy.

Questions to ask at my next checkup

- Is my blood pressure normal?
- Can I keep playing sports or exercising the way I used to do?
- I have not felt my baby move yet. How do I know she is okay?
- If I have had a cesarean section before, must I have one this time?

Other questions I have:

1. _____

2. _____

*Heartburn:
A burning feeling in your chest that is common in pregnancy. It has nothing to do with your heart. It is caused by liquid from your stomach going back up into the tube connecting your mouth and stomach.

■ ■ ■ ■ ■ ■ ■ ■ ■ ■

Tip–What to do about heartburn?*

Try eating many small meals and chewing your food well. Wear loose clothing. Sleep with your head and chest raised about six inches. Stop eating any foods that make your heartburn worse. If these things don't work, ask your provider what medicines you can take safely to help you feel better.

My four-month checkup

On this date, _____, I had my four-month appointment.

I am ____ weeks pregnant.

I weigh ____ pounds (kilos) now.

I have gained ____ pounds (kilos) since my last checkup.

I have gained ____ pounds (kilos) since I got pregnant.

My blood pressure is _____.

Things I learned today

1. _____

   _____

2. _____

   _____

My next checkup will be on

the _____ of _____, at ____:____.
    (date)   (month)   (time)

■ ■ ■ ■ ■ ■ ■ ■ ■ ■

Tip–Swollen legs: Do your legs and your feet swell when you stand up for a long time? Try:

- wearing support hose,
- putting up your feet when you are sitting,
- moving around often,
- standing with one foot up on a low stool or box,
- wearing flat shoes that have plenty of room for your toes,
- eating fewer salty foods and drinking fewer diet sodas.

Shape up for pregnancy...

These exercises help your body stay strong through your whole life.

1. "Kegel squeeze" helps birth muscles

This exercise (named for Doctor Kegel) strengthens the muscles around the opening of your vagina. **Those muscles hold up your growing uterus. They also must be able to relax and stretch open during delivery.** The exercise also helps hold your vagina and bladder in place as you get older. It even may help you enjoy sex more!

An easy way to learn this exercise is while you are urinating on the toilet. Here's how:

- Squeeze your vaginal muscles to stop or slow the flow of urine. Try **not** to tighten your stomach muscles or buttocks.

- Hold tight while you count 1–2–3–4–5.

- Relax, and then squeeze again. (After you know how this exercise feels, don't do it while urinating.)

Your pelvis tilts when you arch your back and pull in your buttocks.

You can do the Kegel squeeze anywhere. **Try it standing at the kitchen sink or waiting for the bus.** Practice until you can do it 25 times, three or four times a day.

2. "Pelvic tilt" lessens low back pain

Strengthening the stomach muscles (see pictures) helps prevent low back pain.

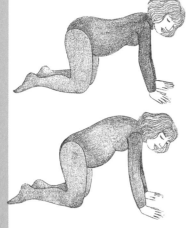

- On hands and knees with your back straight, breathe in and relax your back.

- Breathe out, tighten your stomach muscles and pull your buttocks under you. Your back will arch. Count to five. Then breathe in again and relax your stomach.

- Now try it standing up. Tighten your stomach and pull your buttocks under. Repeat this as often as possible each day.

...And for later life

Here are two other easy ways to shape up your body now and later.

3. Standing straight and tall

Standing with your back very straight can lessen low back pain. It also helps you look slim and feel good about yourself. To see how this looks, do it in front of a long mirror.

- Stand sideways to the mirror with bare feet. Pull your chin in and your head up.

- Bring your shoulders down and back. Pull your belly in and your buttocks under. This is like doing the Pelvic Tilt.

See how your belly and buttocks look smaller. Feel how your muscles work together. Practice standing and walking this way. Soon it will become a habit.

4. Squatting and sitting cross-legged

These two ways of sitting loosen your hips and the joints of your pelvic bones. They also stretch your inner thighs. **Both can help with back pain now. They also will help when you are pushing your baby out during birth.**

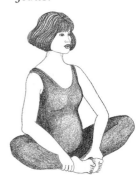

Squat holding onto a chair for balance to stretch your pelvic joints.

- To squat, start with feet apart. Hold onto a chair so you do not fall. Squat down, keeping your heels on the floor, if possible. (Don't try this if you have knee problems.)

- Sit cross-legged on the floor. Spread your knees wide apart and cross your ankles. For more stretch, put the soles of your feet together.

For more stretch while sitting on the floor, put your feet together.

79

Keeping the loving feeling during pregnancy

You both may find that your enjoyment of sex is changing. As your belly grows larger, sex may be less enjoyable. However, some women find it more exciting. Your partner may have different sexual feelings, too.

You can try new ways to enjoy sex. Tell your partner what positions feel best now. Try lying on one side, with your partner behind you. Many women find that position the easiest when their belly gets very big.

There are many ways to enjoy being together. Talk about the kinds of touches that feel good to you. At times, just being close and holding each other can be enough. This is an important time to talk about what you are thinking and feeling.

Remember that sexual feelings are likely to return after you heal from giving birth.

Having sex will not harm your baby if your pregnancy is normal. It does not make labor start. Sometimes, however, the doctor or midwife may tell you not to have sex. Sex could be harmful to the baby's health if you are having bleeding or after your waters have broken. (See page 116.)

If any bleeding or water comes from your vagina, stop having sex. Call your doctor or nurse-midwife for a checkup. Any time you have questions, be sure to ask your provider.

It is still important to protect yourself from sexually transmitted diseases. Both partners must get treatment if either one has an STD. This is essential to an unborn baby's health.

■ ■ ■ ■ ■ ■ ■ ■ ■ ■

Tip–Painful breasts: As your breasts grow larger and heavier, they may hurt. A firm bra that fits well will keep them as comfortable as possible.

My fifth month (19 to 23 weeks)

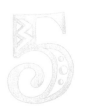

How is my body changing?

- You will now be gaining about 3 to 4 pounds (1300 to 1800 grams) each month.
- The top of your uterus may be up to your belly button.
- The skin on your face may get light or dark patches. A dark line may run down the middle of your belly. These changes will disappear after pregnancy.
- You will probably have plenty of energy and feel very well this month.

How is my baby growing?

- At the end of this month, your unborn baby will be up to 12 inches long (30 centimeters). He is more than half as long as a newborn baby.
- He will weigh almost one and one-half pounds (680 grams). This is about as much as a large loaf of bread.
- His skin is very wrinkly. It is covered by a thick white coating called "vernix."
- He moves enough now for you to feel his kicks easily. He also has rest times.
- Hair is starting to grow on his head.

■ ■ ■ ■ ■ ■ ■ ■ ■ ■ ■

Tip–A birth helper: If you have not already done so, find a birth partner. You may want more than one helper.

Some people may find birth very hard to see. Your baby's father may not want to take part in the delivery itself. He needs your understanding if he feels that way.

What can I do to stay healthy?

- Go for your regular checkups.
- Continue to stay away from cigarettes, alcohol, or any drugs.
- Walk to different places (the store, the park) so you don't get bored. Invite a friend along for company.
- Be sure to drink eight glasses of liquids each day.
- Eat plenty of healthy foods, like vegetables, beans, whole wheat breads, and yogurt. Save sweets for special treats.
- If you have been told to take prenatal vitamins, take them every day.

Questions to ask

- Is my baby growing well?
- How could my job be harmful to my baby?
- Is there any chance I could be having twins?
- Where can I find a good childbirth class?
- How long should I keep on working?
- Is my blood pressure normal?
- What can I do about varicose veins?

Other questions I have:

1. _____

_____

2. _____

_____

■ ■ ■ ■ ■ ■ ■ ■ ■ ■

Tip–Buckling up: Use your lap and shoulder belts every time you ride in a car. Push the lap belt down below your belly and pull it tight. Keep the shoulder belt snug over your shoulder and between your breasts. (See page 42.)

My five-month checkup

On this date, _____, I had my five-month appointment.

I am ____ weeks pregnant.

I weigh ____ pounds (____ kilos) now.

I have gained ____ pounds (____ kilos) since my last checkup.

My blood pressure is _____.

Things I learned today

1. _____

   _____

2. _____

   _____

3. _____

   _____

My next checkup will be on

the _____ of _____, at ___:___.
   (date)   *(month)*   *(time)*

■ ■ ■ ■ ■ ■ ■ ■ ■ ■

Tip–Preventing constipation:

- drink about 2 quarts of water (8 to 10 glasses) a day,
- get exercise every day,
- eat foods with plenty of fiber, like fresh fruits and vegetables, prunes, brown rice, and whole wheat breads,
- eat some dried prunes every day,

Your doctor or nurse-midwife may recommend a stool softener if you get constipated.

Looking ahead: How will I feed my baby?

This is the time to start thinking about how to feed your baby. You do not have to decide right now. Here are some things to think about:

Breastfeeding gives babies the best start!

- Breast milk gives your baby all the food she needs for the first 6 months.

- **Both colostrum* and breast milk give your baby antibodies* that protect her from illness.** She will probably have fewer allergies, ear aches, colds, diarrhea, and other problems.

- Breastfeeding can help you and your baby feel very close.

- Breastfeeding costs nothing. However, you must eat nutritious foods, drink lots of water, and get plenty of rest.

- Breast milk is always ready and always the right temperature. You can feed your baby almost anywhere.

- The size of your breasts does not matter for breastfeeding.

- You can pump your breast milk into a bottle. It will keep in the refrigerator for up to 24 hours. Freeze it to keep it longer. This way, father or others can feed your baby.

Make sure your health care provider checks your nipples now. If you have inverted nipples (see picture at left), you can wear breast shields before birth (lower picture). The shield will help pull the nipples out so they fit into your baby's mouth.

Some people may try to talk you out of breast-feeding. Many mothers today have not tried it and do not know how well it works.

More about breastfeeding on pages 133 - 134.

*Colostrum: Yellowish liquid made by a woman's breasts during the last months of pregnancy and the first few days after birth.

*Antibodies: Cells made in the body to fight diseases.

Inverted, flat nipple goes in when squeezed.

Breast shield can help nipple come out.

Bottle feeding your baby

Bottle feeding can work very well, too, if you decide not to breastfeed. Millions of babies grow up happy and healthy this way. (See page 135.)

(See page 135.)

- When you or your partner hold your baby to feed him, you can feel very close.

- **You should use formula* for your baby, not cow's milk.** Cow's milk from the grocery store does not have the right nutrients for a baby. It is not easy for babies to digest and should not be used until babies are one year old.

- Formula is made to be like breast milk. However, it does not have your antibodies to fight illness. Many babies who are fed formula have more illnesses in the first year.

- Formula comes as a liquid or a powder. Follow the directions to mix it. Many doctors and nurse-midwives suggest formula with iron.

- You will need to buy bottles and nipples. They must be washed very well after each feeding.

*Formula: Special milk for bottle-feeding; made to be as much like breast milk as possible.

Tip–Give breastfeeding a try:

It's a wonderful start for your baby. You can switch from breast to bottle if you need to, but not from bottle to breast. Your breasts stop making milk after birth if your baby does not suck on them.

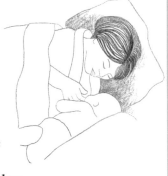

If you have trouble getting started with breastfeeding, ask for help right away. There often are very simple ways to make it easier. A Lactation Specialist,* a La Leche League counselor, or a WIC nurse can help you while you are learning to breastfeed.

Many doctors and nurse-midwives advise mothers to breastfeed for nine months or more. However, breastfeeding for a few months or weeks is better for your baby than not doing it at all.

*Lactation Specialist: a nurse trained to help with breastfeeding (lactation).

85

When labor begins too soon

Sometimes labor starts too early, before 37 weeks. This is called preterm labor. It can be very harmful to the unborn baby. Often, labor can be stopped to give the baby more time to grow. Every day a baby spends in the uterus helps him be more ready for life outside.

It is important to know the signs of preterm labor. These signs do not always mean you have preterm labor. However, it is best to call your health care provider right away in case you need special care. Let your provider decide!

Warning signs of preterm labor

Call your provider right away if you have **any** of these signs:

- bleeding or pink or brown fluid coming from your vagina
- loss of the mucus plug or clear water leaking from the vagina
- contractions every 15 minutes or less, or cramps like those during menstruation
- low back ache that may be steady or come and go
- heavy feeling in your pelvis and vaginal area, like the baby is going to fall out
- unusual tightness or hardness of your belly
- a general feeling that something is wrong

Some women are more likely to have preterm labor than others. If you are expecting twins, are under stress, or have had any of the problems listed on page 13, talk with your doctor or nurse-midwife. You may be asked to take special care of yourself and be monitored at home. Monitoring lets your provider know right away if labor begins.

My sixth month (24 to 27 weeks)

How is my body changing?

- The top of your uterus is now above your belly button.

- You may feel your uterus getting hard and tight, then relaxing. These are normal "Braxton-Hicks" contractions.* They mean your uterus is getting ready for labor.

- You will probably have a good appetite now.

- You may get stretch marks on your belly and breasts. Your belly may itch as your skin stretches. (Lotion may help stop the itching.) Your navel may pop out.

- Your legs may get cramps at night and your ankles may swell.

*Contractions: The tightening of the muscles of your uterus. You will feel your belly get hard and then relax.

How is my baby growing?

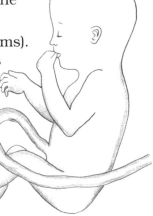

- At the end of this month, your baby will be up to 14 inches (35 centimeters) long. That is about the length of your arm from elbow to fingertips. She lies curled up, her knees against her chest.

- Your baby will weigh about 2 pounds (900 grams). This is as much as a quart of milk (a little less than a liter).

- Her eyes are almost completely developed. Her eyelids open and close.

- She can hiccup and suck her thumb.

■ ■ ■ ■ ■ ■ ■ ■ ■ ■

Tip–Talking to your baby: Soon your baby will be able to hear sounds from outside the uterus. He may learn the sound of your voice. You could tell him how you are getting ready for his birth.

What can I do to stay healthy?

- Keep eating many kinds of healthy foods. Fish, chicken, liver, lentils, and beans are important for your baby's growth.
- Keep away from people who are smoking. Put off drinking beer or wine until after birth and breast-feeding are finished.
- Sign up for a childbirth class.
- Join a prenatal exercise group if you have a hard time exercising by yourself.
- Take some time to have fun with friends before your baby comes. Try a picnic in the park, a movie, a quiet dinner together.
- Remember to buckle your seat belt whenever you ride in a motor vehicle. Pull the lap belt tight. Push it down under your belly. Keep the shoulder belt snug across your upper body.

Questions to ask at my next checkup

- Should I try breastfeeding?
- Am I likely to go into preterm labor?
- Why do I feel my baby move often on some days and less on others?
- How do I know if I am getting enough exercise?

Other questions I have:

1. _____

2. _____

■ ■ ■ ■ ■ ■ ■ ■ ■ ■

Tip–Diabetes in pregnancy: Some women get diabetes while they are pregnant (gestational diabetes). This can cause serious problems for mother and baby. Most women are tested for this disease at about 26 weeks. If you have it, you can learn to control it. It usually goes away after birth.

My six-month checkup

On this date, _____, I had my six-month appointment.

I am ____ weeks pregnant.

I weigh ____ pounds (__ kilos).

I have gained ____ pounds (__ kilos) since my last checkup.

My blood pressure is _____.

Things I learned today

1. _____

   _____

2. _____

   _____

3. _____

   _____

My next checkup will be on

the _____ of _____, at ____:____.
     (date)   *(month)*   *(time)*

■ ■ ■ ■ ■ ■ ■ ■ ■ ■

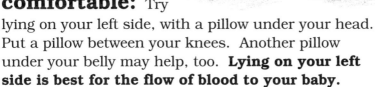

Tip–Getting comfortable: Try
lying on your left side, with a pillow under your head. Put a pillow between your knees. Another pillow under your belly may help, too. **Lying on your left side is best for the flow of blood to your baby.**

Things your baby will need

Clothes

❏ **Tee-shirts, sleepers with legs, socks, a warm hat.** Start with the 6-month size. Most babies outgrow the smaller sizes very quickly. If your baby is born early and is small, he could use newborn clothes at first.

❏ **Diapers:** Which kind is best? There are benefits and problems with each kind. A diaper service or disposable diapers can be easy to use but usually cost more than washing your own.

Furniture

*Car safety seat: A special kind of seat for use in motor vehicles. Also called a "car seat" or a "child restraint."

❏ **A car safety seat*** that fits a new baby. (See the next page.) You should use it on every ride. Start with the trip home from the hospital.

❏ **A place for your baby to sleep** with a firm mattress, sheets, and blankets. At first, you could use a cradle or a box. Later you will need a bigger crib with solid sides or narrow spaces, 2 3/8 inches (6 cm) or less, between the bars. **Beware—older cribs with wider bar spaces could catch a baby's head.** Some have other safety problems, too.

Supplies

❏ **For you: nursing bras**, large enough for your breasts filled with milk. These open in front to make breastfeeding easier.

*Non-aspirin pain reliever: Medicine made without aspirin, used to lessen both fever and pain. "Tylenol" is one brand. **Aspirin can be harmful for babies and young children.**

❏ **Bottles, nipples, and formula**, if you do not plan to breastfeed.

❏ **Medicines that babies may need**. These include "non-aspirin" liquid pain reliever* for fever and ointment for diaper rash. Ask your doctor or nurse about medicines you should keep at home.

❏ **A thermometer**. A regular thermometer is fine, unless your health care provider asks you to take your baby's temperature rectally. In that case, you need one with a rounded end. (See page 145.)

How do I choose the "best" car seat?

Buckle your baby into a car safety seat. Car crashes hurt or kill many children every year. Laws in all states of the U.S. and in Canada require young children to be in car safety seats on every ride. Your hospital will expect you to use one for your baby.

Car seats can be very hard to understand and use right. For help, see the Purple Pages, page153.

The "best" car seat is the one that fits your child and vehicle and that you can use right on every trip. There are two kinds for babies:

1. **Small car seats for infants only,** weighing under 20 to 22 pounds (picture). Do not use a household infant seat, which will not protect in a crash. Infant-only seats are:

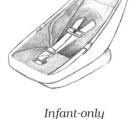

- Lightweight, easy to carry from car to home.

- Low in cost, but when the baby outgrows it you must get a larger seat.

2. **Convertible safety seats** fit babies and children up to 40 pounds, about age 4. These face the rear for infants up to age one and at least 20-22 pounds, then can be turned to face forward.

Infant-only car seats fit newborns well and are convenient to use in home and car.

- A seat with harness only (see lower picture) fits newborn babies better than a seat with a shield. A seat with a padded shield attached to shoulder straps fits larger babies.

- Some hold a baby rear-facing to 25-30 pounds.

Before choosing, try the seat in the car:

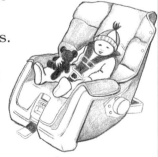

- Make sure the safety seat fits in your vehicle facing the rear. **If the car has a passenger-side air bag, always put your baby in the rear seat.** The air bag can kill a baby!

- The safety belt fits around it and holds the seat from sliding forward or from side to side. Read the instructions for both seat and vehicle and try it.

Larger convertible car seats with harness fits children from birth up to 40 pounds.

Ask your hospital, clinic, or auto insurance company about low-cost car seats. Beware—second-hand car seats may have serious safety problems.

Other things you and your baby may enjoy

❏ **A baby tub** for easy, safe baths. A foam cushion helps keep your wet baby from slipping.

❏ **An infant feeding seat.** Your infant car safety seat can be used in the house, too.

❏ **A rocking chair or a baby swing.** The rocking motion makes most babies feel happy and peaceful.

❏ **A cloth baby carrier** for holding your baby close when you go for walks. You can keep your baby with you and have your hands free. When your baby is fussy, try carrying her in this inside the house. It will probably calm her.

❏ **A pacifier** for your baby to suck on. Sucking can calm a fussy baby, but not all babies or parents like pacifiers. Baby's thumb is a natural pacifier. If you want to try using a pacifier for your baby, make sure it is all one piece of rubber. Look for the kind that is shaped to fit a baby's mouth. Be sure not to tie it with a string around your baby's neck. The string could strangle him.

❏ **Baby toys** that are soft and washable. Toys should not have small hard parts that your baby could chew or pull off. These could choke a baby. Avoid long strings that could get wrapped around her neck.

*Mobile: A pretty toy that hangs down and moves in the breeze. Babies like the shapes, the colors, and the motion.

❏ **A mobile*** to hang high over your baby's bed. Get one with bold black and white or brightly colored shapes. These will be easiest for your baby to see. Look up at it to make sure the shapes will show from your baby's position.

❏ **Books and pamphlets** on taking care of babies. Look for these at your clinic or doctor's office. See the Purple Pages for other places to find helpful information.

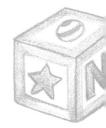
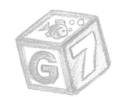

Chapter 6

Months 7 and 8

28 to 35 weeks

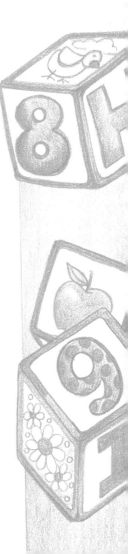

Your third trimester (months 7, 8, and 9) is starting. Your pregnancy is almost over. You have done a lot to help your baby be healthy. Are you eager to get started being a parent?

This chapter is short because it covers only two months. Chapter 7 includes both the ninth month and birth. **Look ahead now at Chapters 7 and 8. They will give you a good start on birth and caring for your newborn baby.**

See the Purple Pages at the end of the book for other places to get information on birth and parenting. A baby care class at the local hospital can be a big help. Take one now if you can. After delivery, you probably won't have time.

If you have other children, tell them about the baby inside your body. Let them feel your belly when your baby is moving. Let them talk to the unborn baby. If you plan to move them into other bedrooms, do it a few months before the baby is born.

Most important: know the signs of preterm labor (page 86). Your baby's health depends on keeping him safely inside your uterus until he reaches about 40 weeks. Call your health care provider right away if you think labor is starting!

Choices about labor and delivery

There are choices that you can make that will help your delivery go the way you want it to. What you learn in childbirth class will help you choose. Now is a good time to read Chapter 7 to find out what happens during birth.

If your labor is going well, you will be able to decide many of these things:

- What **positions to use during labor and delivery:** standing, walking, sitting, or squatting may be more comfortable than lying on your back.
- What ways you would prefer to use to cope with **pain.** (See page 114.)
- If you want to **breastfeed right after birth**.
- If your partner will **cut the cord**.
- Whether to **have your baby stay in your room** or in the nursery.
- If you have a boy, will he be **circumcised**? (This surgery cuts away the loose skin around the tip of the penis.) (See page 99.)

Think these things over during the next three months. **Talk about them with your provider, your baby's father, and your childbirth teacher**. Make sure your doctor or nurse-midwife knows what you prefer.

If problems come up, your doctor or midwife may not be able to follow all your wishes. For example, having twins or premature labor could change your plans. If things must be done differently, be sure you understand why.

Maternity leave

This is also the time to plan for maternity leave from your job. You will need some time to recover from birth. You and your baby also need time to get to know one another. If you are breastfeeding, you may want to stay home for the first six months.

94

My seventh month (28 to 32 weeks)

How is my body changing?

- You could gain another 4 pounds (1800 grams) this month.

- Your bulging belly may make you feel awkward. Your hip joints are getting looser and may ache. This also can make you feel clumsy. You may feel dizzy when you stand up suddenly.

- You may feel kicks against your ribs. You will be able to see your belly bulge as your baby moves.

- You may feel hot and may sweat more than usual. Wear light, loose clothing to stay cool.

- Colostrum may leak from your breasts.

How is my baby growing?

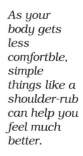

- At the end of this month, your baby will be up to 16 inches (40 centimeters) long. He will weigh about 4 pounds (1800 grams).

- His body is well formed. He would have a good chance of surviving if he were born now.

- You may feel him hiccup. He can even suck his thumb!

If you are having twins or multiples, watch for signs of preterm labor. (See page 86.) Avoid having sex or orgasms that could make labor more likely to start.

As your body gets less comfortble, simple things like a shoulder-rub can help you feel much better.

Tip–practice your exercises:

Exercises are more important than ever in the next few months. Practice the pelvic tilt, Kegel squeeze, and standing straight. (See pages 78-79.) Take time every day to squat or sit on the floor cross-legged. Also do your breathing exercises. **These will help you feel more comfortable now and have an easier birth.**

What can I do to stay healthy?

- Go to your prenatal checkups.
- Go to your childbirth classes and encourage your birth partner to go with you.
- Drink at least 8 glasses of water every day.
- Do gentle exercises like walking.
- Be sure to rest every day. Lie on your left side with a pillow between your knees or sit with your legs up on a chair.

Questions to ask at my next checkup

- How long should I plan to keep working?
- Am I likely to go into labor early (preterm labor)?
- Do I have inverted nipples?
- I eat lots of vegetables, fruit, and grains but still get constipated. What should I do now?
- Should I count how often my baby moves?

Other questions I have:

1. _____

   _____

2. _____

■ ■ ■ ■ ■ ■ ■ ■ ■ ■

Tip–Baby care: Learn as much as you can now. This is especially important if your health plan usually sends new moms and babies home soon after delivery. Three ways to learn:

- Go to new-parent classes at the hospital or birth center before your baby is born.
- Watch a video on infant care. Ask your health care provider for one.
- Spend time with other new mothers and babies.

My seven-month checkup

Today, _____, I had my seven-month appointment.

I am ___ weeks pregnant.

I weigh ____ pounds (__ kilos).

I have gained ____ pounds (__ grams) since my last checkup.

My blood pressure is _____ (see below).

Things I learned today

1. _____

_____

2. _____

_____

My next checkup will be on

the _____ of _____, at ___:___.
    (date)   *(month)*   *(time)*

Warning–High blood pressure: High blood pressure (pregnancy-induced hypertension or PIH*) during pregnancy can become dangerous to you and your baby. If your provider finds your blood pressure is high, you will need to take special care of yourself to prevent more serious problems.

The signs listed below may mean that PIH is getting worse. You may need emergency care, so call your provider right away!

- sudden weight gain (more than a pound per day)

- headache

- swelling of hands and face

- blurred vision or spots before your eyes

- nausea and vomiting

*Pregnancy-Induced Hypertension: Sometimes called PIH, preeclampsia, or toxemia. A serious disease that happens most often to women having their first baby.

Choosing your baby's doctor

*Pediatrician:
A doctor who
has several
years of
special
training in
the health
care of
children.

Your baby will need a family physician or pediatrician* to see that she is healthy and stays that way. It is important to find one before birth.

If your provider is not a family physician, ask her to recommend doctors. Check with your health plan for the providers on its list. Then meet the providers yourself. Questions to ask before choosing:

- Does she have an office or clinic either near your home or easy to get to? Do the office hours fit your schedule? You will go there often for checkups.

- Is he friendly and easy to talk to, with time to answer questions? Does he have a nurse who can give you advice by phone when you need it?* (Your health plan may have an information line.)

**If you are
deaf or hard-
of-hearing,
you may want
a health care
provider who
has tty
service.*

- Is she easy to reach in an emergency? Does she have other providers you can call when she is away?

- Do his concerns match yours? Some parents have strong opinions about certain child health issues.

- Is the care affordable? Is she on the list of your insurance plan?

***Pediatric
Nurse-
practitioner:**
A nurse with
special
training in
children's
care, who
works with a
family
physician or
pediatrician.

Babies and children need to see their doctor or nurse-practitioner* regularly even when they are not sick. Usually babies have about six "well baby" checkups in their first year.

Try to avoid using the emergency room for minor illnesses. That care is expensive. Also, the doctor or nurse there does not know your child or her history.

How will I pay for my baby's care?

If you have health insurance for your family, the plan will cover new babies. **Call the plan soon after birth to tell them about your new child**.

If you have no insurance, call your public health department or community clinic. These places can help you find care for yourself and your baby.

My eighth month (33 to 36 weeks)

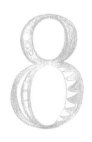

How is my body changing?

- You will probably gain about 4 more pounds (1800 grams) this month.

- The top of the uterus is getting up to your ribs. You may have trouble breathing when your baby pushes against your lungs.

- Your hands and feet may swell.

- Your body may feel very warm. Light, loose clothes will help.

- You may need to urinate often, even at night, because your baby is pressing on your bladder.

How is my baby growing?

- Your baby will grow to about 18 inches (45 centimeters) in length, and will weigh about 5 pounds (2200 grams).

- He can open his eyes and see light.

- He may move less than last month. There is less room to turn over inside the uterus now.

- Your baby will settle into one position in the uterus. He may be head down or buttocks (bottom) down.

- Your belly will bulge when the baby pushes on it. Can you feel the head, feet, and elbows?

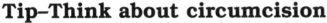

Baby's uncircumcised penis

Tip–Think about circumcision

now: If your baby is a boy, do you want him circumcised? This is a choice for you and your baby's father to make together. Circumcision is usually done soon after birth. There is no clear medical need to do it, but you may have religious, family, or personal reasons.

Circumcised penis

What can I do to stay healthy?

- Go to 2 checkups this month.

- Keep up your healthy habits. Stay away from alcohol, drugs, and cigarettes.

- Take time to take a walk every day, even if you move more slowly now. Practice the exercises you learn in your childbirth class.

- Be sure you are eating plenty of foods rich in calcium—dry beans, milk, tofu, peanuts, dark green vegetables.

- Put your feet up whenever you sit down.

- After you choose a doctor or clinic for your baby's care, be sure to tell them.

Questions to ask at my next checkup

- Is my baby growing well?

- Can my partner and I still have sex and what positions are best at this time?

- Is my baby lying head down or head up?

- I sometimes leak urine when I cough or sneeze. Does this mean something is wrong?

- Is it healthy to keep exercising as I get closer to delivery?

- Should I register at the hospital or birth center before I go into labor?

  Other questions I have:

  1. _____

  _____

  2. _____

  _____

Review signs of preterm labor: Read
page 86 again to remind yourself of signs to look for.

My first eighth-month checkup

On this date, _____, I had my first eight-month appointment.

I am ____ weeks pregnant.

I weigh ____ pounds (___ kilos).

I have gained ____ pounds (___ kilos) since my last checkup.

My blood pressure is _____.

My baby's position: _____.

Things I learned today

1. _____

   _____

2. _____

   _____

My doctor or nurse-midwife wants me to call when I have these signs of labor:

1. _____

2. _____

3. _____

4. _____

My next checkup will be on

the _____ of _____, at ____:____.
   (date)   *(month)*   *(time)*

■ ■ ■ ■ ■ ■ ■ ■ ■ ■ ■

Tip–Talk to your baby: Remember, your baby can hear the sounds you make. Does he ever move when he hears sounds from beyond your body? Tell him how you are getting ready to be his parent. Tell him about his family.

Especially for father

Getting ready for baby's birth

This is a page to show your baby's father, if he has not read the whole book!

You are essential to your unborn baby's life, birth, and growth. Here are some things to do as you wait for birth.

- **Feel your unborn baby move** by putting your hand on your partner's tummy.

- **Talk to your baby** about things you will do with him after birth.

- **Go to checkups** with your partner.

- **Go to childbirth classes** and practice the breathing exercises with her between classes.

- **Help pick out the baby's car seat.** (See page 91.) Learn how to use it correctly. (See page 136.) Read the directions and practice putting it in the car. This is a very important way to keep your baby safe.

- **Talk about names** you like for your baby.

- If you think you do not want to see the birth, say so. You could help during labor and leave the room when the birth takes place. **You can be a good father without seeing your baby born.**

- **Sex will not harm your unborn baby**, unless there has been bleeding, the bag of waters has broken, or your partner is having preterm labor. She may not feel much like having sex in the weeks before and after birth. Talk with her about what positions are comfortable for her. Ask her what kind of touching she would like.

If you feel left out by your partner at this time, tell her. She may think about her unborn baby most of the time. Being able to tell each other how you are feeling is a healthy habit.

Take time together to do things that will be harder after your baby is born. Visit friends. Take a few days off for a vacation. Go to the movies. Get plenty of sleep!

My second eighth-month checkup

On this date, _____, I had my second eight-month appointment.

I am ____ weeks pregnant.

I weigh ____ pounds (___ kilos) now.

I have gained ____ pounds (___ kilos) since my last checkup.

I have gained ____ pounds (___ kilos) since I got pregnant.

My blood pressure is _____.

Things I learned today

1. _____

_____

2. _____

_____

3. _____

_____

My next checkup will be on

the _____ of _____, at ____:____.
   (date)   (month)   (time)

■ ■ ■ ■ ■ ■ ■ ■ ■ ■ ■

Tip–Your baby's movements:

Pay attention to how often your baby moves. Babies have quiet and active times each day. But babies usually move at least 10 times in 12 hours. Count your baby's kicks and punches. **Call your health care provider right away if you think your baby has slowed down or stopped moving** for two or three hours.

Let your other children feel your baby move. Help them talk to their unborn brother or sister, too.

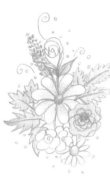

The big day is almost here!

Whether your pregnancy has been easy or not, you know it will end soon. You will soon have a new child to love. You have already started to be a parent by taking care of your unborn baby.

What names are you thinking of giving your baby?

_____

_____

_____

_____

How do you feel now?

____ Excited

____ Scared

____ Happy

____ Depressed

____ A little bit of all of these

Other feelings? _____

_____

What are your special hopes?_____

_____

_____

Do you have new concerns now? _____

_____

_____

Share how you feel with your partner or husband, or with a close friend.

Chapter 7

Month 9: The Birth Month

36 to 40 weeks

The ninth month brings an end and a new beginning. Birth is the welcome end of pregnancy. It is the start of parenthood. Labor and delivery are natural events that may seem strange and surprising. **To start getting ready, read this chapter before your ninth month.**

This chapter has notes about your ninth month checkups. It also gives you the main facts about birth. To be completely prepared, you will need to know more. The more you learn now, the less surprised or scared you will feel during birth.

A childbirth class is the best place to learn about your birth choices. It is important to learn about these choices, so you can share your desires with your doctor or nurse-midwife. If you have not been able to take a class, be sure to talk with your provider.

You or your birth partner should not be shy about asking questions during your labor and delivery. Sometimes things you had not expected may be happening. Your provider may have to do some things that you did not want. Make sure you understand why these things are needed before they are done.

How is my body getting ready for birth?

Braxton-Hicks contractions are the way your uterus gets ready for real labor. They are painless and get stronger as delivery gets closer. These "practice" contractions usually stop when you move around.

When you feel your uterus getting tight and hard, you can practice special ways of relaxing. Childbirth classes teach breathing methods and other ways of relaxing. These are all ways to help the contractions do their work.

During the ninth month, you will have a checkup each week. Your doctor or nurse-midwife will tell you if your baby has "dropped." This means the uterus has moved down between the pelvic bones. This is one of the first steps toward birth. You may see that the bulge of your belly is lower.

Next your cervix will start to efface (thin) and dilate (open). Your health care provider probably will check your cervix each week. She can tell you how it is changing.

*Mucus plug:
Thick, gooey matter fills the opening of your cervix during pregnancy. It keeps germs from getting inside the uterus and harming the baby.

The mucus plug* that has filled the cervix will come out as the cervix changes. Watch for this thick blob and tell your provider. It may have a little bright red blood with it. It is also called "bloody show."

No one can tell ahead of time when your labor will begin. Your baby and your body will start labor when they are ready. Some women's bodies show clear changes in the last month before labor begins. Others do not.

Labor usually begins any time from two weeks before your "due date" to two weeks after it. Labor may take a few hours or many hours. Your first birth is likely to take longer than later ones.

Turn to page 115 to find out what happens during birth. The signs of labor are listed on page 116.

Your ninth month (36 to 40 weeks)

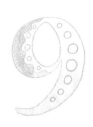

How is my body changing?

- You will probably gain about 4 more pounds (1800 grams) in this month.

- Some time this month, the baby will drop into your pelvis. Breathing and eating may be more comfortable after this happens, but the baby will press harder on your bladder and rectum. You may need to urinate more often. You also may get more constipated.

- You may feel very tired. It is normal to feel this way. Give yourself time to rest.

- Just before labor begins, you may feel new energy. This is a good time to pack your bag with things to take to the hospital or birth center. (See page 110.) Try not to get tired out. You will need your strength for birth.

How is my baby growing?

- Your baby is getting heavier. Most babies are about 20 inches (50 centimeters) long at birth. Most weigh about 7 pounds (3200 grams) or more.

- All the parts of her body are well formed now. She could be born any time.

- Her fingernails are getting longer.

- She has grown to fill the uterus and has little room to move. She may seem quieter.

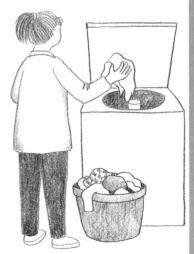

■ ■ ■ ■ ■ ■ ■ ■ ■ ■ ■

Tip–Help after birth: Find some friends or family members who will be able to help around the house for the first few weeks. Some of the most helpful things they can do are laundry, dishes, and shopping. You can spend your time and energy with your new baby.

What can I do to stay healthy?

- Be sure to eat prunes, whole wheat bread, fresh fruits, and vegetables. These help to keep your bowels moving.
- Do your relaxation and breathing exercises.
- Get plenty of rest, with your feet up.
- Learn as much as you can about labor and delivery. This is a good time to read the rest of this chapter.
- Go for your checkups each week.

Questions to ask at my next checkup

- How will I know if my contractions are real labor? When should I call you?
- What positions (sitting, squatting, or lying down) may work best during labor?
- If I need pain medication, what kinds might you use? How would they affect me and my baby?
- Who can I turn to for help with breastfeeding?

Other questions I have:

1. _____

   _____

2. _____

   _____

3. _____

   _____

■ ■ ■ ■ ■ ■ ■ ■ ■ ■ ■

Tip–Registering at the hospital:

Call the hospital or birth center and ask how to register ahead of time. That would make it easier for you to be admitted when you arrive in labor.

My first ninth-month checkup

On this date, _____, I had my first nine-month appointment.

I weigh ____ pounds (____ kilos) now.

I have gained ____ pounds (____ kilos) since my last checkup.

My baby has dropped? Yes ___ No ___

I am ___ percent effaced* or ___ centimeters dilated.* (This may not be measured at every checkup this month.)

My baby's position is head down ___ or bottom down ___.

Things I learned today

1. _____
   _____

2. _____
   _____

My next checkup will be on

the _____ of _____, at ____:____.
$\quad$ (date) $\qquad$ (month) $\qquad$ (time)

*Effaced: A measure of how thin the cervix has become. This happens after the baby drops and as the cervix opens.

*Dilated: A measure of how far the cervix has stretched open. (See page 119.)

■ ■ ■ ■ ■ ■ ■ ■ ■ ■ ■

Tip–Getting to the hospital: Plan

who will take you to the hospital or birth center. Make sure the person taking you knows how to get there. If you have never been there, go once to learn the way. Have a second person ready to drive you in case the first driver cannot do it.

If you have other children, make sure you have one or more people who will be able to take care of them.

What should I pack for the hospital?

❏ **This book!**

❏ **A watch with a second hand**. Your partner can use it to know how long contractions last and how often they come.

❏ **A radio or tape player** and your favorite tapes. Soft, quiet music can help you relax during labor.

❏ **A camera** to record the birth. If you want this, make sure you have film. Test the camera ahead of time to make sure it is working properly.

❏ **Sugarless candies** to keep your mouth moist.

❏ **Nightgown** that opens in front for nursing, robe, slippers, and warm socks.

❏ **Hairbrush**, toothbrush, toothpaste, makeup. Leave jewelry and money at home.

❏ **Nursing bras** that open in front, a bed jacket or sweater, underpants. You will need menstrual pads (not tampons) if the hospital does not give them to you.

❏ **Snacks** for your birth partner and for you after birth. Prunes, nuts, whole-wheat crackers, and apples will help keep your bowels moving. They also will be more tasty than most hospital food.

❏ **Clothes for you to wear home.** Take something loose. Your body will not be as slim as before you got pregnant

❏ **Clothes for your baby** to wear home, like a one-piece sleeper with legs. Add a hat and thick blanket if the weather is cold.

❏ **The car seat** for your baby's first ride home. You and your baby should ride buckled up, even in a taxi. If you do not have a seat by now, ask if the hospital lends them. (Buckle it into the car so it will be ready for your trip home.)

What you will need to know at the hospital

These are things you will need to know when you get to the hospital or birth center.

Fill out this part early this month

❑ Blood type (ask your doctor or nurse): _____

❑ Your doctor or nurse-midwife's name:

_____

Phone number:_____

❑ The name of the doctor or nurse-practitioner who will care for your baby:

_____

Phone number:_____

❑ What kinds of pain relief would you prefer if necessary? _____

_____

❑ Do you plan to breastfeed? ____ Do you want to breastfeed right after birth? _____

❑ If your baby is a boy, do you want him circumcised before he goes home? _____

Fill this in when contractions have begun

❑ How many minutes between the start of one contraction and the start of the next?

_____

How many seconds do they last?_____

❑ Has your bag of waters broken already? _____
If so, when and what color was the liquid?

_____

❑ Do you have discharge from your vagina? _____
If so, what color is it? _____

My second ninth-month checkup

On this date, _____, I had my second nine-month appointment.

I weigh ____ pounds (____ kilos) and have gained ___ pounds (____ kilos) since I got pregnant.

I am ___ percent effaced and ___ centimeters dilated (if measured).

Things I learned today

1. _____

2. _____

My next checkup will be on

the _____ of _____, at ____:____.
     (date)   *(month)*   *(time)*

Questions for my next checkup:

1. _____

2. _____

■ ■ ■ ■ ■ ■ ■ ■ ■ ■ ■

My third ninth-month checkup

On this date, _____, I had my third nine-month appointment.

I weigh ____ pounds (____ kilos) now.

I am ___ percent effaced and ___ centimeters dilated (if measured).

Things I learned today

1. _____

2. _____

My next checkup will be on

the _____ of _____, at ____:____.
     (date)   *(month)*   *(time)*

My fourth ninth-month checkup

On this date, _____, I had my fourth nine-month appointment.

I weigh ____ pounds (____ kilos) now.

I am ___ percent effaced and ___ centimeters dilated (if measured).

Things I learned today

1. _____

2. _____

How I am feeling now

_____

_____

After birth, you can keep a record of what happened on page 125.

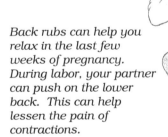

Back rubs can help you relax in the last few weeks of pregnancy. During labor, your partner can push on the lower back. This can help lessen the pain of contractions.

■ ■ ■ ■ ■ ■ ■ ■ ■ ■ ■

Tip–If your baby is late: Your baby is not really "late" until two weeks after his due date. This may seem like a very long time to wait, but remember, no one is pregnant forever! If you have not started labor one or two weeks after the baby was due, be sure to talk with your doctor or nurse-midwife about the action she thinks is best.

Questions about labor and birth

During labor, your nurse-midwife and the nurses will have many practical tips. They have helped many women through labor. Make sure they know the kind of birth you hope to have.

Do relaxation, breathing, and massage help?

Yes, you will have less pain if you can relax. Special breathing and massage are two ways to do this. Your birth partner can help you to breathe properly. He or she can rub your belly lightly or massage your back.

It will be easier to relax in a quiet, peaceful room. If people in the hall or visitors distract you, you can close the door or ask people to wait outside.

What position will be best for me?

Not every mother goes through labor lying down. Other positions may help you feel more comfortable. They also can help your birth go quicker or easier. If you are sitting or standing, the baby's weight will help pull it down into the birth canal.

These are some positions to try:

- standing or walking
- resting on hands and knees
- squatting and leaning back with support

Will I need pain medication?

You may not need medication or want it. You may want the full experience of birth and your labor may be going well. Relaxation, special breathing methods, and changing positions may be enough.

However, if labor is very long or contractions are very hard, drugs can bring relief. Different kinds are used depending on your condition and how far along in labor you are. Learn about these before labor begins. See the next page for more.

What kinds of pain medication might I have?

- **Pain relievers**, like Demerol: you can feel the contractions, but they will not seem as painful.

- **Tranquilizers** may help if you are very nervous and other relaxation methods have not worked.

- **A spinal or epidural** numbs certain parts of the body; you cannot feel contractions.

Your health care provider will weigh the risks and benefits to mother and baby. He also will take your wishes into account. Discuss this before birth.

Ask your provider about the kinds of drugs she prefers to use and why. **Any drug may have side effects on you and your baby.** It is important to know the risks before you are given a drug.

What will birth be like?

These are the stages of birth:

1. **Labor** contractions make the cervix thin and dilate completely.

2. **Delivery** of the baby by pushing with the contractions.

3. **Delivery** of the placenta.

4. **Recovery** of your body's strength and shape.

Early labor—your cervix starts to open

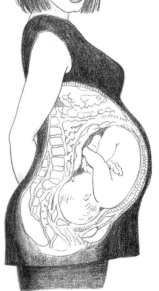

In the last few weeks before the birth, the uterus drops (sinks down) between the pelvic bones. Contractions press the baby down into the cervix. They make the cervix dilate (open) and efface (get thinner). This happens earliest with first babies.

Most babies are born head first (see picture). Others come out bottom first (breech).

Before labor begins, the uterus drops down between the pelvic bones. The cervix is beginning to thin and open.

115

How will I know if labor has started?

Here are some signs of labor that your body may give you. You may not have them all.

- ❏ **Contractions that get longer and come closer and closer together.** They get stronger when you move around. Write down on page 120 how long they last and how often they come. Your doctor or nurse-midwife will want to know this.
- ❏ Pain that moves from your lower back around to your belly.
- ❏ Several soft bowel movements.
- ❏ The mucus plug (bloody show) coming out of your vagina.
- ❏ Clear liquid gushes or leaks from your vagina when the amniotic sac breaks. Your water may break a few hours or a day before labor starts or only after it begins.

False labor

Sometimes it is hard to tell if the contractions you feel are "the real thing." You may be having false labor if:

- Contractions do not get stronger when you get up and walk,
- Pain is only in the lower part of your belly.

If you are not sure, call. Your doctor or nurse-midwife will not mind being called at any time. Sometimes the only way to know if true labor has started is to be checked by your provider. She can tell how much your cervix has effaced and dilated.

Making labor start (inducing labor)

Sometimes it is necessary for your provider to induce labor using drugs. This is often done if labor has not started by two weeks after the due date. It can also be done if serious problems come up earlier.

When should I call my doctor or midwife?

Remember the signs your doctor or nurse-midwife has told you to watch for. (See page 101.) If you are not sure when to call, do so when:

- **your bag of water breaks**

- **your contractions have come about 5 to 10 minutes apart for an hour.**

Tell your provider as much as you can about what is happening to your body.

Call any time, day or night. It is better to call early rather than wait too long. You may be told to stay at home for a while longer. This is most likely if this is your first birth.

Getting to the hospital or birth center early does not help labor go faster. But if you live far from the hospital, be sure to call early.

Good things to do for yourself

These are ways to stay comfortable and help labor go well both at home and at the hospital or birth center.

- Stay at home until your doctor or midwife says to come to the hospital or birth center.

- Eat lightly if you think you are starting labor. Have thin soups, fruits, and crackers instead of a large meal.

- Drink water or juice, or suck on chips of ice.

- Urinate every one or two hours.

- Change positions often during labor. Walk around, sit up, stand, kneel on hands and knees, or squat.

- Rest and relax. Save your energy for the hard work ahead.

117

Tips for a birth partner

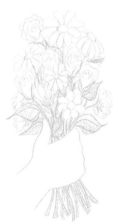

Here are ways to help, both at home and after you get to the hospital or birth center.

- **Keep calm** and cheerful. Help your partner breathe and relax during contractions.

- Time her contractions so she will know what progress she is making. (See page 120.)

- Play her favorite tapes or a radio softly if music relaxes her.

- **Keep the room quiet** while your partner is having contractions. If other people are there, ask them to leave the room for a while. This is not a time for visiting.

- **Encourage her to change positions** or walk around. Even if she doesn't want to move, it could help her be more comfortable.

- Light or firm massage can help relax her during contractions. Press on her lower back firmly if it aches.

- **Urge her to rest** between contractions. Help her breathe calmly during the contractions.

- You may feel strange seeing your partner's body working hard in the later part of labor. It is normal for her to have nausea and pain. She may cry, groan, or be grouchy. Remind her that the hardest part will be over soon.

- If the doctor or nurse-midwife thinks your partner needs some medication or other help, ask why. **Make sure you both understand why something different is to be done.**

- If you feel tired, take a little time away by yourself. Leave the room, get a snack, or go outside into the fresh air for a few minutes. You will be more able to help if you are not exhausted.

As a father, you play a very important part of the birth of your baby. Being there to welcome your child into the world is very special. This is true even if you choose not take part in the whole birth.

If you are a friend, you probably will always have a special feeling for this baby.

Contractions

Your cervix opens wide

Your body can do amazing things! At the time of birth, the uterus is the largest and strongest muscle in your body. When it contracts, it first pulls your cervix open. Then it pushes your baby out.

Labor means that your uterus is working to dilate the cervix. You cannot stop these contractions. Instead, you need to relax and let the uterus do its work.

How your cervix opens during labor:

- **Early labor**: Contractions are short and not too strong. Your cervix opens to 4 centimeters. You can do your normal activities during this time.

- **Active labor**: Longer and stronger contractions come closer together. During this time you should go to the birth center or hospital.   Your cervix will open to 8 centimeters.

- **Transition**: When the cervix dilates completely, to 10 cm. (4 inches). This is wide enough for your baby's head. Contractions now are hardest, strongest, and come closest together.

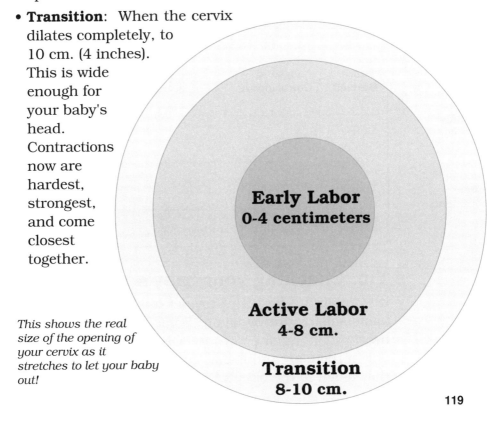

This shows the real size of the opening of your cervix as it stretches to let your baby out!

Early Labor
0-4 centimeters

Active Labor
4-8 cm.

Transition
8-10 cm.

119

Keep track of your contractions

The length and frequency of your contractions tells you and your provider how your cervix is dilating. Use a watch with a second hand to time your contractions. Use the chart below.

Phase	cm. dilated	length (seconds)	frequency (minutes)
Early labor	0-3 cm.	30-45 sec.	15-30 min.
Active labor	4-7 cm.	45-60 sec.	3-5 min.
Transition	8-10 cm.	45-90 sec.	2-3 min.

Write below the exact time when a contraction begins. Note when it ends. Its **length** is the number of seconds it lasts. Note when the next one starts. The minutes or seconds between the start of one and the next is the **frequency**, how often it happens.

Also note below the time when other things happen. The waters may break during this time, for example.

* Signs such as water breaking and color of the water, bloody mucus, bowel movements.

Your Contractions

Time Started	Length of Contraction	Frequency of Contractions	Other Signs*
_____	_____	_____	_____
_____	_____	_____	_____
_____	_____	_____	_____
_____	_____	_____	_____
_____	_____	_____	_____

Continue on another sheet of paper

Tip: Checking your baby's heartbeat

It is important for your provider to know how your baby is doing during labor. Some hospitals use fetal heart monitors for everyone. Others use monitors only if there are problems. Instead, in normal labors, they listen to the baby's heart with a doppler.

Delivery: When the baby is born

After the cervix is completely open, you will probably feel like pushing. Pushing with the contractions will move the baby down the birth canal and out. See the pictures on the next page.

Stretching your perineum

Your vagina and perineum* must stretch wide to make way for the baby's head. You may have a burning feeling as the head presses against the skin.

*Perineum: The skin and muscles around the opening of the vagina.

Your doctor or nurse-midwife may tell you not to push too hard for a little while. She may hold her hand on the top of the baby's head to slow down delivery. This gives the perineum time to stretch. Warm or hot towels or gentle massage may also be used to avoid tearing or the need for an episiotomy.* However, if your provider feels it is necessary, an episiotomy may be done.

*Episiotomy: A short cut made in the perineum to prevent tearing as the head comes out.

Sometimes, if a baby's head is not coming out as it should, a doctor may use forceps to gently pull it out. Sometimes a vacuum extractor is used.

After the head has been born, the rest of your baby's body comes out very rapidly. You will feel a great relief that delivery is almost over! Your baby may be placed right on your abdomen or wrapped up to keep warm while you hold her.

After birth: The placenta is born

The delivery of the placenta, sometimes called the "afterbirth," will seem easy. Your uterus will contract a few more times. You may need to push a little more to help the placenta come out.

Now your provider may massage your uterus or give you medication to help it get firm. This can be uncomfortable. The uterus should stay firm to limit bleeding. If you had an episiotomy or tear, it will be sewn up. Finally, you can relax and enjoy your baby.

A baby's vaginal birth

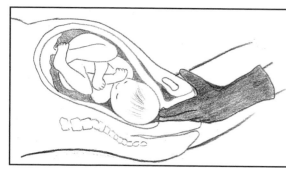

The first stage: Labor

The cervix has thinned out and opened. The baby starts to move into the vagina. In most cases he will be born head first.

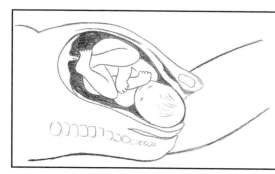

The second stage: Delivery

Now the baby's head has reached the opening of the vagina. The skin around the vagina must stretch slowly so it does not tear. If it does not stretch enough, an episiotomy may be done.

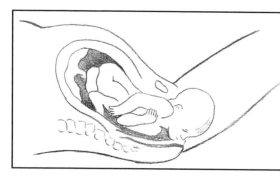

The baby's head has appeared. The shoulders come next. After that, the rest of the body comes out very quickly.

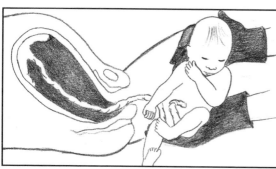

Now the newborn baby begins to breathe and is checked quickly. The umbilical cord will be clamped and cut.

The third stage follows:

The placenta, still in the uterus, will be delivered after more contractions.

Possible problems at birth

Cesarean delivery (C-section)

A cesarean delivery* is done through a cut in your uterus through the belly. It is quite common, yet may be done more often than necessary. It is more risky for the mother than a vaginal birth, and recovery takes longer.

A C-section is usually done when certain problems come up during birth. Some reasons are:

- The baby is lying bottom down instead of head down.
- The baby is too large to fit through the pelvis.
- There are problems with the umbilical cord or placenta.
- Mother or baby has a known health problem that makes a vaginal birth unwise.
- The baby is not doing well during labor.

Many women can have a vaginal birth after having had a cesarean (called VBAC). If your scar goes across your belly, not up and down, it is possible. Your health care provider will know as your labor progresses if vaginal birth will work.

*Cesarean delivery: The baby is delivered through a cut made in the belly and uterus. Medication is used so the mother feels no pain. Also called a "C-section."

Preterm birth

A baby born earlier than 37 weeks is called preterm or premature. Twins and multiple births often come early. (See page 86.)

Babies born very early may not have developed enough to live outside the uterus or to be healthy. A premature baby needs extra care after birth. Yet today, many very tiny premature babies grow up to be healthy people.

Low birthweight babies

Some babies born after 37 weeks are smaller than usual, under 5½ pounds (2500 grams). These babies may be small because they have other health problems. They often need special care. Again, with good care, most grow up to be healthy people.

Welcome your new baby!

After the uncomfortable contractions and hard work of pushing, your new baby has come into the world.

Your baby may look strange to you at birth. He will be wet, and his skin will be a blue-purple color. He may be covered with white vernix and streaks of blood. He may seem lifeless for a moment, but after his first breath he may cry. **His lungs are taking in air for the first time. His skin color will start to turn to its natural color.** The doctor or nurse-midwife may suck mucus out of his nose and mouth to help him breathe better.

The **umbilical cord** will be clamped and cut now. This separates your baby from your body. Your birth partner may be able to cut it if he wants. Cutting the cord does not hurt you or your baby.

Your baby's general health will be checked quickly one minute and five minutes after birth. Your doctor or nurse-midwife will look at his heart rate, breathing, muscles, body reflexes, and skin color. He is given an "**Apgar score**" between 1 and 10. (Ten is the highest score.) You may want to note the score on the next page to remember it.

It is important to keep your baby warm. He will be dried right away and wrapped in a blanket. **Then he will be given to you to hold against your skin or put under warm lights. You may be able to breastfeed now.**

This can be a very emotional time. Some women may feel overwhelming love for their babies right away. Others can't believe birth has really happened. Some may wonder if they can take care of such a small person. It is normal to have any or all of these feelings at this time.

You or your partner may want to write notes about your baby's birth on the next page. This will help you remember this special day.

My Baby's Birth Day!

My baby's name is _____

Baby was born on _____ (date)

　　at _____ time in the morning __ or night __.

Weight: ____ pounds (____ grams)

Length: ____ inches (____ centimeters)

Head circumference (distance around): ____ inches
(____ centimeters)

First sign of labor: _____

Date and time when I arrived at the hospital or birth
center _____

I was in labor for _____ hours.

Things I did that helped labor go well

_____

Pain medication I was given, if any

_____

Special things done by my doctor or nurse-midwife
to help deliver my baby

_____

_____

Apgar Score at 5 minutes after birth _____

How I felt right after birth _____

_____

Comments by my birth partner _____

_____

Comments by my doctor or nurse-midwife

_____

_____

125

What happens next?

Now that your baby is born, you finally can see and hold him or her. What an exciting time! Take some time to hold your baby close right after birth. Most newborns are wide awake for about 1 to 2 hours after birth. Then they need a long sleep.

If you plan to breastfeed, you will probably want to start right after birth. The colostrum in your breasts gives her a good start. Let her feed while she is alert. This is a way to get off to a good start with breastfeeding.

If you had a vaginal birth, don't be surprised if your baby's head and nose look oddly shaped. This is from being squeezed through the birth canal. They will return to their normal shape in a day or two.

Soon after birth, your infant will be given an injection of vitamin K to prevent possible bleeding problems. Medicine will be put in her eyes to prevent infection. It may make her eyes red for a day or two.

Your nurse-midwife or hospital nurses will help you start to feed and care for your baby. **Nurses are good teachers. Ask them any questions you have.** Also read the next chapter.

Coming home

If both you and your baby are doing well, you will probably come home within a day or two after delivery. If you have had a cesarean delivery you will stay longer to recover. If your baby is small or had problems at birth, she will probably stay longer, too.

A home nursing visit can be very helpful to new parents. If your hospital or health plan does not offer you this service, ask if it is available.

Your health care provider, your baby's doctor or nurse-practitioner, and the hospital or birth center all have people who can help you, day or night.

Chapter 8

Caring for Your New Baby

Birth to 6-8 weeks

Your newborn baby can do amazing things! Both you and your baby's father will learn this as you watch and listen to him. **See how he tries to tell you what he wants.**

He can see your face when you hold him close (8 to 10 inches away). He likes looking at faces, lights, red objects, and black and white patterns.

He can hear sounds and knows your voice. Babies like the high, sing-song sound of "baby talk." Don't feel silly talking this way—it's natural. Hold him against your chest so he can hear your heart beat. He knows this sound from being in the uterus.

Your New Baby's Reflexes

A new baby has many reflexes. These automatic reactions show how well he is developing. They will disappear later.

- He will hold on tightly to your finger.

- When he hears a loud sound he will be startled. His arms and legs will straighten suddenly.

- If you stroke his cheek he will turn his head and open his mouth.

- When he is on his tummy, he will move his arms and legs as if he is crawling.

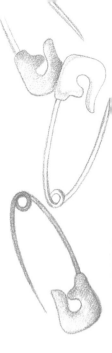
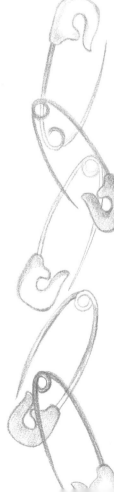

127

Holding your baby

Your newborn baby's head is heavy and her neck is weak, so keep your hand or arm under her head. You can hold her up to your shoulder, cradle her in one arm, or hold her under your arm.

Never shake your baby in fun or anger. This could seriously damage her weak neck and her brain. Rough bouncing or swinging also could injure her.

Caring for a baby with a special need

Does your baby have a birth defect or another health problem, like low birth weight or prematurity? If so, he will probably need to stay in the hospital for a while for special medical care.

Both you and your baby's father can help care for him in the hospital. Your baby needs to hear your voices and feel your touch. Visit him often so you will know how to care for him at home.

If your baby has a birth defect

If your child has a birth defect, it may be a shock at first. Parents whose baby is not born exactly the way they expected may feel very frightened, sad, and angry. These feelings are normal. Here are some ways to cope.

- Spend as much time as possible with your baby.

- **Talk with the hospital social worker.** She can be a great help. Partners may need support from professionals and other parents to get through this time. The social worker can link you with a parent support group.

- Ask for a second opinion if you are not sure about approving any treatment.

Modern medical care helps many babies with defects to lead healthy, happy lives. Your baby will need your love and attention. **Caring for him can be very hard and very special at the same time.**

128

Your new baby and your family

Enjoy being a new father

As a father, you are very important in your baby's life. As a man, you bring your own special kind of parenting to your child.

Take time, right from birth, to touch, cuddle, and talk with your newborn baby. She will learn quickly to know your voice, smell, and touch. When she is wide awake, hold her close and talk to her quietly.

Take some time to care for your baby all by yourself. Learning to diaper and bathe her will give you both time to get to know each other. You can learn your own way to be a parent.

Your older children

Your other children may not find your new baby as exciting as you do. She will take most of your attention. **Your other children may have some sleep, toilet, and behavior problems for a while.** Here are some tips.

- Plan to spend some special time with each older child every day. Let them know you still love them just as much as before.

- Let older children help you with baby care, but stay with them at all times. They may not understand that they could harm the baby. For example, a child may be eager to hold her but not be able to cradle her head properly.

- Do not leave the baby alone with a child under age 10. A baby is too much responsibility!

Tip–Twins, triplets, or more: If you have had twins or triplets, you and your partner almost certainly will need as much help from friends and family as you can get. Look in the Purple Pages in this book for the mothers of twins group. It can give you useful advice.

Your baby will start changing right away. See the last page of this chapter for changes you may see by the end of the first month.

129

Understanding your baby

Don't worry if you do not know all about baby care. You will learn as your baby grows and changes. Treat your baby gently and ask any questions you may have. See page 152 for places to get help.

Your newborn baby can't talk, but she does try to let you know what she wants. If you, your baby's father, and other caretakers try to understand, you all will get along better. Listen and watch your new baby's face and body.

- **When your baby is sleepy**, her eyes will blink open and closed. She will move her arms and legs slowly and make quiet noises. Her body may jerk when she hears loud sounds.

- **When your baby is in a deep sleep**, she breathes evenly and does not wake up easily.

- **At times she may sleep more lightly.** Her breathing will be less regular and you may see her eyes move. She may suck with her mouth and move her arms and legs slowly.

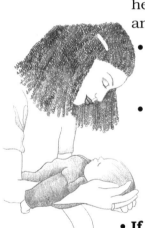

- **When she is waking up** she may not be ready to eat or play. Talk to her, rub her body, change her diaper. Give her time to wake up.

- **When she is awake and alert**, she is busy learning about the world. She will look at you and listen to your voice. A newborn baby can only do this for a minute or two at a time. Then she will look away or turn her head. That's a sign that she needs to rest.

- **If your baby is tired and fussy**, she may try to help herself feel better. Putting her hand to her mouth is one way she does this. Give her time to relax. Hold her close and rock her quietly.

- **Crying is the way she asks for help.** She may be hungry or in pain. Crying may also comfort her if she is very tired.

When your baby is awake and alert, she will look at your face eagerly.

Tip–Playtime: Playing with you helps your baby learn. Hold her close to your face while she is alert. Talk softly to her. Watch her reach out her arms toward your face. She may try to copy the expression on your face or make a noise at you.

What to do when your baby cries

Do you feel upset when your baby cries? That is normal for new parents. **But crying is a natural way for your baby to tell you something.** It may mean he is hungry, tired, wet, lonely, uncomfortable, or sick. You and your baby's father will soon be able to tell his hungry cry from his tired cry.

Many young babies have a fussy time every day, often at night. This is called colic. They feel better after they cry for a while, but parents get upset because they are not be able to comfort them. Most babies outgrow colic by 3 months of age.

Cuddle and rock your baby as much as he wants. ***This will not spoil a young baby.***

Some ways to comfort a fussy baby:

- Change his diaper if it is wet or dirty.

- Let him suck on your clean finger or a pacifier.

- Wrap him snugly in a blanket (swaddling).

- Hold your baby and rock him to sleep.

- If he has been awake for a while, he may be very tired. He may need to cry for a few minutes in his crib before he can sleep.

- Put your baby in a carriage or front pack and walk with him in the house or outside.

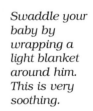

If he is acting very different from usual and you cannot comfort him, check if he has a fever or other signs of being sick. (See page 146.) If he does, call your doctor or nurse-practitioner.

Swaddle your baby by wrapping a light blanket around him. This is very soothing.

If your baby cries often and you can't soothe him, **some foods may be bothering him**. Talk to his health care provider about this. Some breastfeeding mothers avoid foods like onions, cabbage, or even milk. A formula made without cow's milk may help.

If you get very upset by your baby's crying, it may be best to put him in his crib to cry for a short time. This gives you time to get over being angry. If this happens often, find an adult you trust to baby-sit. Avoid taking alcohol or drugs when you are upset. Your baby is not trying to make you mad.

Feeding basics

Feeding time is a special time for parent and baby. It is a quiet, soothing time for feeling close.

It is best to feed your newborn when she is hungry, not on a schedule. (If you have twins you may have to feed them on more of a schedule.) New babies who breastfeed are often ready to eat every 1½ to 3 hours. Babies who are bottle-fed may be hungry every 3 to 4 hours.

A baby's appetite will change from week to week. When your baby is growing faster, she will need to have more breast milk or formula or to eat more often. Feed her when she shows signs of hunger.

Usually a baby who is hungry makes little sounds and sucks on her fist. She will turn her head toward your breast if you are holding her. If she does not get fed, she will start to cry hard.

Is your baby getting enough to eat?

A baby under 4 to 6 months of age should get enough food from the breast or bottle if he feeds when he is hungry. Check to make sure she:

- **Has at least 6 wet diapers every 24 hours** and has soft bowel movements.

- Gains weight after the first week (she may lose some at first).

- Becomes sleepy or calm after eating and burping.

Burping gets the air up

Often a baby will need to burp in the middle of a feeding and at the end. Hold her on your shoulder, across your knees, or on your lap. Pat or rub her back gently. Some milk or formula may come up when a baby burps. This is normal. Don't forget to use an extra cloth diaper to protect your clothes!

Note: If your baby vomits hard, so liquid shoots several feet out of her mouth, call your baby's provider right away!

132

Starting to Breastfeed

Breast milk is the perfect food for babies. Most babies are able to breastfeed right after birth. For the first few days, your breasts will make nutritious colostrum. Then they start to produce breast milk.

Breastfeeding may not "come naturally" to you at first. Once you get started, it can be a very happy time. Almost any woman can breastfeed with help.

Ways to hold your baby while you breastfeed:

- Lying in bed on your side. Your baby rests on the mattress or in the bend of your elbow.

- Sitting in an armchair, hold your baby in the bend of your arm. Put a pillow under your elbow and rest it on the arm of the chair.

- Holding your baby under your arm with his feet behind you. This is the most comfortable way if you have had a cesarean delivery.

Baby's position is key to happy breastfeeding

There are two things to check to help keep your nipples from getting sore:

- **Baby's tummy must face your body.** If he has to turn his head to reach your nipple he will pull on and twist the nipple.

- **He must latch on to both the nipple and areola** (dark area around the nipple). Your baby's mouth squeezes the glands inside the areola to suck milk out. Sucking the nipple does not work.

Three steps to help him latch on correctly:

1. Hold him so his tummy is facing yours.

2. Hold your breast in your hand and touch his lower lip with the nipple.

3. When he opens his mouth wide, pull him toward your breast. Guide the nipple and areola straight in. Watch to make sure he gets all or most of the areola into his mouth.

Some medicines and drugs and germs can pass to an infant through breast milk. Check with your health care provider before taking anything.

Hold your breast with your fingers below and your thumb above the nipple. Help him take the nipple and areola into his mouth so it points straight in.

133

More breastfeeding hints

If you breastfeed your baby, be sure to eat well. You will need plenty of protein, liquids, and calcium. Turn back to pages 34 - 39 for more on nutritious food.

- When your breasts first begin making milk, your breasts may get "engorged" (hard and painful). **Breastfeeding as often as possible at the start will help prevent or limit this problem.** Warm cloths will help make the milk flow easier. Engorgement usually lasts only a few days.

- Your areola may get so full that your baby can't get it into her mouth. Express (squeeze) a little milk out by hand to make it softer. Stroke your breast firmly with your fingers, from the sides toward the areola. Then squeeze and release the areola with your thumb above and fingers below.

- If your nipple does not stand out, you can roll or pull it between your fingers before feeding.

- **Your breasts make just enough for your baby's appetite.** When she sucks more, they will make more milk. They can make enough to feed twins!

  - Switch breasts half way through each feeding, after about 10 minutes, or when her sucking slows. Start each feeding with the breast she ended with the last time.

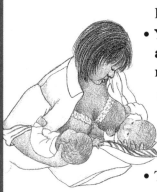

Nursing twins at one time.

- To get her to let go of the nipple, put your finger gently into the corner of her mouth. This will break her suction without hurting your nipple.

- **Let your nipples dry in the air after feeding**. This helps prevent soreness.

- Ask your baby's doctor or nurse-practitioner if your infant needs extra vitamin D or fluoride.

Get help for problems right away

***Lactation specialist:** A nurse with special knowledge of breast-feeding.

If you are having problems, ask for help right away! **Don't just stop breastfeeding or wait until it gets worse.** Call your doctor or nurse-midwife or a lactation specialist.* A local La Leche League group (see page 152) can give you practical advice and support. You also can turn to these people to help you breastfeed when you go back to work.

Bottle feeding your baby

Hold your baby in your arm against your chest while you feed him. Look at him and talk softly. **It is important for you to hold him.** He needs this time to be close to you. **Do not prop up the bottle.** He could choke lying alone with the bottle.

Put the nipple straight in. Tip the bottle up so the nipple is not full of air. Some nipples are shaped to fit a baby's mouth. Ask your health care provider what shape she suggests.

Holding your baby close helps him feel loved. He should feed reclining in your arms, not lying flat.

Hints about bottle feeding

- Use formula with iron unless your baby's health care provider tells you not to. Cow's milk is not healthy for babies under age 1.

- If your formula has to be thinned, mix it with slightly warm water when you are ready to feed. Follow the directions on the package. Be sure to measure correctly. If the formula is too thin or too thick, it could affect your baby's growth.

- If your water comes from a well or other private source, it may not be clean enough for a newborn. **If you are not sure how clean the water is, use boiled (and cooled) water or bottled water for your baby.** Lead in the water from pipes in old buildings also can be a hazard. (See page 47.)

- Formula should be at skin temperature. Test it by dripping a little onto the inside of your wrist. It should flow out in slow drops.

- While your baby is a newborn, mix only a few ounces in the bottle at one time. Do not force your baby to finish every bottle. **Always throw out what she does not use at a feeding.**

- Use a fresh bottle for each feeding. If you need to warm it, put it in a pan of hot water for a few minutes. **Never heat a bottle in a microwave oven.** The formula can get hot enough to burn your baby, even if the bottle does not feel hot.

135

Coming Home: Buckling up baby

Buckle up your baby on his very first ride, going home from the hospital. Start a good safety habit for every ride. **A car safety seat can save a child's life. But it can only work if it is used every time, and used correctly.**

If you do not have a car seat yet, see page 91. You may be able to rent one in your area.

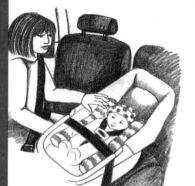

A new baby rides facing the back of the car. Rolled-up towels on both sides keep him comfortable.

How to use a car seat correctly

• Make sure you follow the instructions that came with the car safety seat.

• Put the harness over your baby's shoulders. Tighten the straps so you can slide only one finger under them. If there is a harness retainer clip, put it at armpit level.

• Install the car seat facing the rear of the car. **If your vehicle has a passenger-side air bag*, place your baby in the back seat facing the rear.** If it inflates, an air bag could seriously injure or even kill a baby riding in the front seat.

• Recline the car seat half way back, so your baby's head does not fall forward.

• **Check your vehicle owner's manual** for information on air bags and using safety belts.

• Buckle the safety belt and pull it snug. Many kinds of belts have different ways of staying tight.

*Air bag: A safety device that inflates instantly in a crash to help protect adults. A passenger-side air bag is in the right side of the dashboard. **Check your vehicle owner's manual**.

Other tips on using a car seat for a baby

• Put your baby in a sleeper with feet. This allows the harness straps to go between her legs.

• If the weather is cold, put your baby in and fasten the straps snugly. Then tuck a blanket over the straps. Blankets wrapped under the straps make the harness too loose.

• **Put rolled-up towels or diapers on both sides of your new baby's body** (see picture). They will keep her from slumping. If she is very small, add a small towel under the crotch strap.

Your baby's bowel movements

What goes in, must come out. Every parent must deal with cleaning their baby's bottom, even though it may be unpleasant.

What are a newborn baby's stools* like? Don't be surprised by the first few bowel movements. They will be thick black meconium.* The next few will be greenish. After that they be yellow.

The look of your baby's stools will depend on whether you give him formula or breast milk.

- **Breast-milk** makes a light yellow, soft stool, like lumpy mustard. In the early weeks, a baby may have 8 to10 small movements each day. Later, one stool each day or every few days is common.

- **Formula** makes a tan or yellow, firmer stool (not harder than peanut butter). A baby will often have one or two movements each day.

If the stools get hard and dry, your baby may not be getting enough liquid. If he is sick, he may lose liquid from vomiting or fever. Talk with your baby's doctor or nurse practitioner.

Cleaning your baby's genitals

Always wipe the genitals* from front (closest to the tummy) to back. This keeps germs from stool from getting into the openings of your baby's genitals. Use a clean cotton ball or clean part of the washcloth for every wipe. If your baby boy is not circumcised, don't try to pull the foreskin back.

Caring for a baby boy's circumcised penis:

- If your baby has been circumcised, wash his penis carefully every time you change his diapers. Drip warm water gently over the penis.

- Ask your doctor or nurse practitioner if you need to use ointment on the circumcision. Keep the diapers loose. Lay your baby on his side or back until it has healed. Healing takes about 10 days.

*Stool: Another word for bowel movement.

*Meconium: Material within your baby's bowels before birth, that is passed as the first few bowel movements.

Always wipe your baby's bottom from front to back.

*Genitals: A boy's penis and girls' vulva and urethra (where urine comes out).

Keeping your baby clean

Preventing diaper rash

*Diaper rash: Redness or small bumps on the skin in the area covered by the diaper.

It is easy to prevent diaper rash* if you:

- Change your baby's diapers after every bowel movement and frequently when they are wet.

- Be sure to wash the area with a soft, wet cloth and dry it before putting another diaper on.

- **Let her bottom be bare for a while every day.** Lay her on her tummy on a diaper while she plays. The air helps prevent diaper rash.

  - If your baby gets diaper rash, be sure to change diapers more often. Spread a baby ointment on the rash when you change the diapers.

Caring for the umbilical cord stump

*Isopropyl alcohol: A kind of alcohol used for cleaning wounds, not for drinking. Also called rubbing alcohol.

Clean the stump and the moist area at its base with isopropyl alcohol.* Do this 2 to 3 times a day. Keep the stump dry by folding the top of her diapers below it. It will fall off naturally in 7 to 14 days. **Never try to pull the stump off.** Call your baby's doctor if the skin around it gets red.

Getting ready for the bath

Collect all the things you will need before you start bathing your baby. Have within reach a washcloth, gentle soap, several towels, fresh clothes, and a clean diaper. This is easier than looking for things while she is wet and soapy. **You must always hold onto her in the water. A baby can drown quickly and silently.**

■ ■ ■ ■ ■ ■ ■ ■ ■ ■ ■

Tip–uncircumcised penis care: If your baby has not been circumcised, do not try to pull back the foreskin (outer covering). Just wash the penis. The foreskin may not loosen until he reaches about 3 years of age.

138

Bathing your new baby

If you keep your baby's cord, genitals, and face clean, he needs a bath only every few days. Until the cord has fallen off, it is best to give your newborn a "sponge bath." This will keep his cord from soaking in the bath water. If he has been circumcised, use a sponge bath until his penis has healed, too.

Give your baby a sponge bath on a flat surface (counter, table, or floor) in a warm room. First collect all the things you will need. Have two bowls of lukewarm water, one soapy and one clean, within your reach. Then lay him on a clean towel. Use a washcloth to clean, rinse, and dry one part of his body at a time. **Always keep one hand on him so he doesn't fall.**

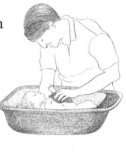

After the cord has healed, wash your baby in a sink or tub with only 2 to 3 inches of warm (not hot) water. Test the water with your elbow. Hold your baby under the head and shoulders with one arm. Soap and rinse with the other hand. **Never leave him alone in the bath—not even for a moment!**

Start bathing him in a small tub after the cord has fallen off.

Dressing for inside and outside

Unless he is very small, **a newborn infant needs to wear only a little more clothing than you do.** Indoors or outdoors, add one layer more than you are comfortable wearing. For the first few weeks, it is best to keep your baby inside if the weather is very cold or hot.

Too many heavy blankets can make your baby too hot. Unless your baby is very low-weight (less than $4^1/_2$ pounds) or is out in cold weather, he probably does not need to be covered with thick blankets.

Your baby will need a hat when he goes outside. In cold weather, babies lose a lot of heat through their heads. In sunny weather, a hat with a brim will protect your baby's face from the sun. **An infant's skin can get sunburned very easily**, so keep him in the shade or lightly covered whenever possible.

Parents' Sleep

Try to take a nap whenever your baby is sleeping. You will need the sleep! Forget all the other things around the house you think you should do.

Baby's Sleep

Many newborn infants sleep most of the time, with short periods awake. Many parents like to have their baby sleep in their room for the first few months.

Your newborn will have periods of deep, quiet sleep and of lighter sleep. While she is sleeping lightly, she may move her arms and legs and make quiet noises. When she is sleeping deeply, ordinary sounds around the house usually will not bother her. You do not need to be very quiet.

When your infant is tired, she will let you know. She will get fussy, turn away, and stop being interested in play. Her eyes will start to blink shut. This is the signal to rock her to sleep or gently put her into her crib.

Sudden Infant Death Syndrome (SIDS) *

*Sudden Infant Death Syndrome: Also called SIDS or crib death. Mysterious death of infants (usually between 1 and 6 months) in their sleep.

No one knows know how to prevent SIDS completely. We know the following things can help lessen the chance of SIDS happening:

- **Baby sleeping on her back.**
- Breastfeeding.
- Mother not smoking, and people not smoking around the baby.

Sleeping on the back is best, so the baby cannot roll onto her tummy. Some parents fear that a baby sleeping on her back could spit up and choke. This has not been found to be true for healthy babies.

Avoid putting soft pillows, fleece pads, and stuffed toys into the crib.

140

Healthy home, safe home

Safe places for your baby

A baby needs safe places to sleep and play. For a newborn, this means places where he can't fall. A crib or changing table with railings or sides will keep him safe. The floor is a safe place to play. Put him on a clean blanket on his tummy to kick and wiggle.

Whenever you change, bathe, or dress your baby on a table, bed, or counter, **keep one hand on his body so he doesn't fall**. Collect all the things you will need so they are in reach before you start.

Cigarette smoke can harm baby

Smoking around a baby can give him health problems. He may have more colds or ear infections, and be more likely to get asthma or pneumonia. Smoke also increases the risk of SIDS. Avoid smoking around him. Ask others to smoke outside when they come to visit.

Avoiding burns

Your baby's skin is very thin and can be easily burned or scalded.

- When holding your baby, avoid holding a hot drink. He could be scalded if it spills.

- When getting the bath water ready, test it with your elbow to make sure it is lukewarm.

- Turn down the temperature of your hot water heater to 120 degrees. That is how to make sure that scalding water never comes out of the faucet.

Smoke alarms save many lives

Smoke alarms in your home are important for your whole family's safety. At least one should be on each level, especially near bedrooms. Change the batteries at least once a year. Your baby's birthday is a good day to change them. Test the alarms every month, too.

Health care for baby

Your baby's health care

Your baby's doctor or nurse-practitioner will check your baby right after birth. In most areas he will check your baby again within a week after you go home. **The provider will ask you to bring her for regular "well baby" checkups 4 to 5 times during the first year.**

Questions about your baby's health and care

It is often hard to remember all the things you want to ask. Write down your questions when you think of them. Take the list to the next checkup.

It also helps to write down the answers when you talk with your baby's provider. This will help you remember all the details later.

Newborn blood tests, immunization

Your baby will have blood tests for a number of serious birth defects. This is done before you leave the hospital or birth center. In many states, all babies get a second blood test (often called a screen) 7 to 14 days later. **If your provider asks you to bring your baby in for a second test, it is important to do so.** This test may find problems that did not show up on the first test.

*Immuniza-tion: A vaccine that builds antibodies in your child's blood. Antibodies fight certain diseases. Most vaccines are given by injection, but polio vaccine may be given by mouth. Also called "shots" or vaccinations.

These tests are for diseases that are not common but could cause serious, lifelong health or mental problems. **Finding and treating them early can prevent or greatly reduce these problems.**

Usually a newborn has her first immunization,* for Hepatitis B, at the hospital. Your baby will get more immunizations at her checkups.

■ ■ ■ ■ ■ ■ ■ ■ ■ ■ ■

Tip–Baby's weight: It is normal for a newborn to lose a little weight right after birth. Your baby should start gaining again within a week.

142

Well-baby checkups

Why does your baby need to see the doctor or nurse-practitioner if he is not sick? Well-baby checkups help keep him healthy. **His provider may find problems you cannot see.** Early care can keep many problems from getting serious. Your baby will get immunizations at checkups, too.

At each checkup, the provider will weigh your baby and measure his length and head size. She will check your baby's ears, eyes, mouth, lungs, heart, abdomen, genitals, hips, legs, and reflexes.

Write down the questions you have before you go, so you won't forget to ask them.

Turn to page 150 (the last page in this chapter) to make notes about your baby's first checkup and immunizations.

Questions _____

_____

Immunizations for babies

Immunizations for babies protect them against ten serious diseases. These are the six vaccines* and the number of doses your baby will need.

- **Hep B** protects against hepatitis B (serious liver infection): three doses by 18 months.

- **DTP** prevents diphtheria, tetanus, and pertussis (whooping cough): four doses by 18 months, one at 4 to 6 years.

- **Polio** prevents polio (called infantile paralysis): three doses by 18 months, one at 4 to 6 years.

- **Hib** (or HBCV) protects against haemophilus influenzae b (which can cause a brain disease): four doses by 15 months (sometimes combined with DTP vaccine).

- **MMR** prevents measles, mumps, and rubella (German measles): one dose by 18 months, one during school years.

- **Varicella** for chicken pox (the newest vaccine): one dose by 18 months. (At this time, not all providers give this to every child.)

*Vaccine: The liquid that is given to immunize a person. Most are given by injection (shots). Some provide protection from more than one disease.

143

Immunizations: gift of health

Why do young babies need them?

It is important to protect your baby by 15 to 18 months of age. This is because many of the diseases are most serious for babies and young children. If your child has a special health care need, she may ger her immunizations at different times.

The diseases that immunizations prevent spread easily from person to person. Before vaccines were discovered, those diseases killed or disabled many people. Today, these diseases are much less common in this country because most people have been immunized. However, outbreaks of measles and whooping cough have happened in the U.S. recently. That is because not all children are immunized.

More about immunizations

After some immunizations, your baby may be fussy and have a low fever for a few days. If the fever goes above 103 degrees, be sure to call your doctor or nurse-practitioner.

It is very rare for a baby to have a severe reaction to an immunization. **If she does not get all her immunizations, she has a much greater chance of getting a serious disease.**

Each vaccine must be given in more than one dose to give full protection. Some must be given again to older children or throughout life.

If your baby misses a well-baby checkup, it is important to go in soon for the immunizations. Immunizations can be given even when your baby has a mild illness like a cold.

■ ■ ■ ■ ■ ■ ■ ■ ■ ■ ■

Tip–Baby exercises: When your baby is awake during the day, put her down on her tummy to play. Watch her push with her legs, try to lift her head, and move her arms.

144

Caring for your sick baby

Before calling the doctor

- Take your baby's temperature if you think he may have a fever. Write down how high it is, how you took it, and the time.

- Make notes of what concerns you. Think about his color, crying, stools, and anything unusual that has happened (like vomiting).

- Have a pencil and paper ready when you call. Then you can write down what the nurse tells you.

- Call your health care provider's office, clinic, or consulting nurse.* The doctor or nurse will also give you ideas about things you can do at home to help your baby feel better. She will ask you to bring your baby into the office if necessary.

Consulting nurse: A nurse who can give you advice when you can't reach your own health care provider.

Taking your baby's temperature

Fever is one sign of illness. You can't tell a fever just by feeling your baby's forehead. Learn how to use a thermometer. Then you can tell his doctor or nurse-practitioner exactly how high the fever is.

Your baby is too young to hold a thermometer in his mouth. You can take his temperature in the armpit, the rectum, or in the ear (with a special tool). Ask your health care provider which way she thinks is best.

Many parents find the armpit is the easiest place to take a baby's temperature. Put the tip of the thermometer in his armpit. Hold his arm against his body for five minutes while you comfort him.

Hold your sick baby close while the thermometer is under his arm.

Using the emergency room

Take your baby to the emergency room only for a real emergency, like a serious injury or illness. Try to call your health care provider first. **Your baby's regular doctor or nurse-practitioner can give him the best care when he is sick.**

Newborn warning signs:

When to call the doctor or nurse-practitioner?

- Temperature under 97.8F (36.6C) or over 100.4F (38C), if not dressed too warmly.

- Forceful vomiting (shooting 2 or 3 feet out of his mouth) or vomiting that continues for more than 6 hours. (Sometimes normal burp may be forceful.)

- Tummy feels very bloated and tight.

- Two or more bouts of green, watery diarrhea, or more than 8 soft bowel movements in 24 hours.

- No wet diapers in 12 hours.

- Refusal to take 2 feedings in a row.

- Discharge or bleeding from any opening (except from the vagina of a newborn girl in the first week).

- Coughing or choking while feeding (except if breast milk or formula is flowing too fast).

- More crying than usual or high-pitched shrieks.

- Bluish skin (except a baby's hands and feet, when they are cold, or his face, when he is crying very hard).

*Jaundice: A yellow tint to the skin that is related to the newborn's liver.

- Jaundice*, the yellowish color of the skin common in the first week after birth, or in the second and third week if you are breast-feeding. Most serious in the first 24 hours.

- Sleepiness, little movement, or a very floppy body.

- Troubled breathing, either fast breathing (more than 60 breaths per minute), very heavy breathing, or no breaths for more than 15 seconds.

- Pus and a red, infected-looking area around cord or circumcised penis.

Call if you see any behavior or look that is not normal for your baby. You will soon learn what is normal for him. If you are worried, it is always best to talk with your health care provider.

146

Taking care of yourself

During the first few days or weeks after birth, you will need plenty of rest and time to get to know your baby. Let others do the housework, or forget it!

What you can expect:

- **Pink or brownish discharge** will come from your vagina for a few weeks. Use pads, never tampons. If you are too active, it may turn bright red again. If you have heavy bleeding or if the discharge smells bad, call your doctor or nurse-midwife.

- **Your uterus will get smaller rapidly.** Your weight will come down too. Use the Kegel squeeze and the pelvic tilt (page 78) to get back in shape.

- **If you had an episiotomy or tear**, your perineum is likely to be sore. Warm baths or pads soaked in Witch Hazel can be soothing. Keep the area clean. Change your pads often.

- **Are you afraid that the stitches will pull out** when you have a bowel movement? Hold some toilet paper against the stitches while you push. Keep stools soft by eating fresh fruits, vegetables, and prunes. Drink about 10 glasses of water a day.

- **If you have trouble urinating**, drink lots of water. Pouring warm water over your vulva while sitting on the toilet may help you get started again. If this doesn't help, talk to your doctor or nurse-midwife.

Eat and exercise for good health

You can help your body heal. Follow the healthy food habits you started in pregnancy. (See page 36.) Walking is an easy exercise to begin with.

Eating right for breastfeeding

While you are breastfeeding, you need to eat healthy foods. Eat plenty of protein and calcium from meat, fish, beans, milk, and cheese.

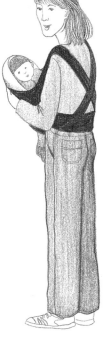

Take your baby out with you in a front-pack.

More on being a healthy Mom

Avoiding alcohol and other drugs

Being a new mother can be hard, but alcohol, cigarettes, and other drugs can make it harder. All of these things damage your health. They can also make it harder for you to handle the hard parts of being a parent.

If you are breastfeeding, these drugs can harm your baby's brain and growth. Breast milk carries alcohol, nicotine, and other drugs to your baby.

Smoke in the air your baby breathes also can give her health problems. Babies of smokers often have more colds, ear infections, and a higher risk of SIDS.

Your own checkups

You should see your doctor or nurse-midwife at least once in the six weeks after birth. He will want to check how your body is recovering and help you decide what kind of birth control is best for you. Be sure to call your health care provider if you have any concerns about your health.

Planning ahead for your next baby

Some women get pregnant again very soon after birth. Most did not plan to do so. **Planning your family means looking ahead and deciding what you and your partner want.** Ask yourselves how many children you want. When do you want another baby?

Did you know?

- **You could get pregnant before your menstrual periods start again.** Breastfeeding may not prevent pregnancy.

- Having your children at least 18 months apart gives your body time to get strong again after birth. It also helps your babies be healthier.

- There are many kinds of birth control to help you plan your family safely and easily.

148

Your feelings after birth

Do you feel sad or moody?

Many women feel depressed for a week or two after they give birth. They may cry easily, feel angry over little things, or have trouble eating and sleeping. This is normal and usually goes away in a few weeks.

These feelings may come from the changes in your hormones after birth. You probably are not getting enough sleep. You may find being a parent a lot more work and less fun that you had dreamed.

Being a parent may seem hard at times, even though you are getting to know and love your baby. Tell your partner, relatives, and friends when you are feeling low. It is okay to say you want time alone with your baby if you have had too many visitors.

If you feel depressed for more than a few weeks, talk to your provider or a counselor. Look for these signs:

- trouble getting to sleep;
- no appetite for food;
- frequent crying, worrying about everything;
- no interest in caring for your baby.

Note: if you start having strange thoughts about hurting yourself or your baby, get help right away!

No one is a perfect parent!

Are you or your partner worried about doing things wrong? You do not have to know all the answers. There are books and videos to turn to. Also, you will feel better as you get more experience.

You and your family can get information from friends, relatives, neighbors, your health clinic, and many organizations. There are parent groups, breast-feeding consultants, and play groups. **Remember, every community has resources to help parents raise happy, healthy children. You do not have to do it alone!**

Every baby is different. You and your partner will both learn from each of your children as they grow up. They will forgive the little mistakes that you may make as you learn to be a parent.

149

Your baby's first 6 to 8 weeks

Newborn Screening

__ first blood screen—probably before going home

__ second blood screen (if required in your state) in the second week

Comments _____

Well-Baby Checkups

The exact schedule will depend on your baby's health and your health care provider or insurance plan.

First checkup   (date) _____

Baby's age ____ weeks;   weight ___ lb. or ___ grams;

Length ___" or ___ cm;   head size ____" or ___ cm

Comments: _____

Date and time of next checkup: _____

First Immunizations   **Dates**

Get a permanent immunization record card and keep it safe.

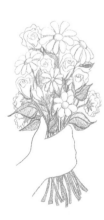

Hep B: first at birth to 2 months   _____

DTP: first at 2 months   _____

Polio: first at 2 months   _____

Hib: first at 2 months   _____

One-Month Milestones

By the end of the first month, most babies are able to:

1. Turn toward a sound.

2. Watch your face as it moves from side to side.

3. Turn her head from one side to the other side when lying on her stomach.

4. Smile sometimes.

Every baby learns at his or her own speed. If you think your baby is developing too slowly, talk with your health care provider.

The Purple Pages

Getting help when you need it

This part of the book is a little bit like the "Yellow Pages" of the telephone book. Here you will find:

- **lists of groups** that can give you help in your community,
- **books** you could read for more details on pregnancy and baby care,
- **telephone numbers** for information lines,
- **a glossary** that gives the meanings of words concerning prenatal health and birth,
- **an index** you can use to find the information in this book.

Inside the back cover is a place for a photo of you and your new baby. I'm glad you have completed your pregnancy, and wish you success as a parent. I hope this book has helped you.

As the author, **I would like to hear any ideas you have on making this book better.** If you have any thoughts, please send them to me at The Willapa Bay Company, 5223 NE 187th St, Lake Forest Park, WA 98155-4345.

If you would like to purchase an individual copy for a friend or relative, please call our office at 1-800-403-1424.

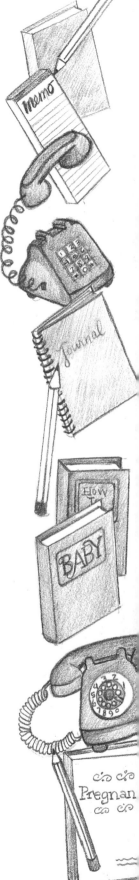

Getting help where you live

You may already know about some of the groups listed here. Others may be new to you. All have useful services for pregnant women and new parents.

Most of the organizations listed have chapters in many cities and towns. Their phone numbers and addresses can be found in the telephone Yellow or White Pages. Look under "Health," "Education," or "Government" listings to find many of them. You can also locate them through your county health department or your hospital social worker.

American Red Cross: Health and safety classes.

ASPO/Lamaze (American Society for Psychoprophylaxis in Obstetrics): Classes in Lamaze method of childbirth preparation and parenting.

Church, synagogue, or other place of worship: Parent support programs.

Crisis hotline: Telephone help and information service for people who are very upset, sad, or angry, including abused women.

Community clinics: Prenatal and well-baby care.

Community college: Parent education for community members.

Community information line: Direct link to local services, available in many cities and counties.

County Health Department: Prenatal and well-baby care and education.

Health insurance Company: Your medical plan may have health or pregnancy telephone information services.

Your health plan: Your health insurance company or HMO may include a health information service.

ICEA (International Childbirth Education Association): Classes in childbirth preparation and parenting.

La Leche League: Information and help with breastfeeding.

Local hospitals: Birth preparation classes, parenting classes.

March of Dimes: Prenatal education and information on birth defects.

More help...

Mental health centers:
Counseling and support groups for people who are having problems.

Parents of Multiples:
Support for families with twins and multiple births.

Parent support groups:
Groups set up by different organizations, where parents support and help one another. Includes groups of new parents, also groups of parents of children with specific disabilities.

Planned Parenthood:
Information and help about birth control and family planning as well as women's health.

Public library: Books, pamphlets, tapes, and notices of educational programs on health.

SafetyBeltSafe USA: Child car safety information and help with problems (see phone number at right).

School nurse: If you are in school, your nurse is a person who is able to help young people deal with new challenges.

Women, Infants, and Children Program (WIC): This effective government program gives healthy foods and health education to pregnant women, nursing women, babies, and young children who qualify.

Numbers to call

Alcohol and drug abuse:
National Clearinghouse for Alcohol and Drug Information
1-800-729-6686

Child abuse:
National Child Abuse Hotline
1-800-422-4453

Childbirth education:
ASPO/Lamaze
1-800-368-4404

ICEA
1-612-854-8660

Domestic violence:
State hotlines or local crisis center hotlines.

Drug abuse:
National Institute on Drug Abuse Helpline
1-800-622-HELP (4357)

Family planning:
Planned Parenthood Federation of America (Smart-line connecting caller with nearest clinic)
1-800-230-7526

Safety of children's furniture and toys:
Consumer Product Safety Commission Hotline
1-800-638-2772

Car seat safety:
SafetyBeltSafe Helpline
1-800-745-SAFE (7233)

National Highway Traffic Safety Administration, Auto Safety Hotline
1-800-424-9393

Choices for further reading

This book has given you the **basic information** every woman needs to know during pregnancy and the first months after birth. You may want to read books that have more details. Here are some books to look for in your library or local bookstores. Planned Parenthood bookstores carry many useful books and pamphlets.

Prenatal Care

A Child is Born, Nilson.

Planning for Pregnancy, Birth and Beyond, American College of Obstetrics and Gynecology, 1990.

Pregnancy, Childbirth and the Newborn, Simkin, Whalley, and Keppler, 1991.

Teens Parenting: Your Pregnancy & Newborn Journey, Lindsay and Brunelli, PHN, 1991.

The Healthy Baby Book - A Parent's Guide to Preventing Birth Defects and Other Long-Term Medical Problems Before, During, and After Pregnancy, Reuben, 1992.

What to Expect When You're Expecting, Eisenberg, Murkoff, and Hathaway, 1991.

Baby Care

Breastfeeding Today - A Mother's Companion, Woessner, Lauwers, and Bernard, 1991.

Caring for Your Baby and Young Child, American Academy of Pediatrics, Shelov, Editor, 1991.

The Parents' Guide to Raising Twins, Friedrich and Rowland, 1984.

The Premature Baby Book, Helen Harrison, 1983

Taking Care of Your Child: A Parent's Guide to Medical Care, Pantell, Fries, and Vickery, 1990.

Teens Parenting - Your Baby's First Year, Lindsay, 1991.

Touchpoints: Your Child's Emotional and Behavioral Development, Brazelton, 1992.

What to Expect: The First Year, Eisenberg, Murkoff, and Hathaway, 1989.

The Womanly Art of Breastfeeding, La Leche League, 1991.

The Year After Childbirth: Surviving and Enjoying the First Year of Motherhood, Kitzinger, 1994.

A Glossary: words to know

Abdomen - The part of your body below your ribs and above your legs. Contains your stomach, uterus, and other organs.

Abortion - Ending of a pregnancy, which may be natural (miscarriage) or done by a doctor (induced).

AIDS - Short word for Acquired Immunodeficiency Syndrome, a fatal disease passed from person to person. Passed most often by having sex or sharing needles. May be passed to an unborn baby.

Air Bag - A safety device for front seat car passengers that is hidden in the dashboard and opens if a crash occurs.

Amniocentesis - A test of the fluid inside the bag of waters, showing certain things about your baby's health.

Amniotic fluid - Liquid in the amniotic sac.

Amniotic sac - The "bag of waters" inside the uterus and in which the baby grows.

Antibodies - Cells made in a person's body to fight disease. A baby's first antibodies come from mother's colostrum and milk.

Aspirin - A drug you can buy without a doctor's prescription that lessens pain and lowers fever.

Areola - The dark area around the nipple.

Bag of waters - The amniotic sac in which your baby grows within the uterus.

Birth canal - Your vagina, the opening through which your baby will be born.

Birth control - Ways to keep from becoming pregnant when you have sex. Examples: condom, diaphragm, pills, IUD.

Birth defect - Baby's health problem that happens before birth or during birth. May have lasting effects.

Blood pressure - The force of blood pumped by the heart through a person's blood vessels. High blood pressure means the heart is pumping extra hard.

Bloody show - A small amount of mucus and blood (the "mucus plug") that comes from your cervix before labor begins.

Braxton-Hicks contractions - Tightening and relaxing of the muscles of your uterus during the last few months of pregnancy.

Breech birth - Birth of a baby buttocks first; much less common than head first.

Calcium - A mineral in foods needed to make bones and teeth grow strong.

Calories - Energy in foods. Some kinds of foods have more calories than others.

Certified Nurse-Midwife - A nurse who delivers babies, who has been specially trained and passed a national test.

Cervix - The neck (opening) of the uterus (womb). Your baby is pushed out through the cervix during delivery.

Cesarean section - Delivery of a baby through a cut through the woman's belly into the uterus.

Child safety seat - A special baby or child car seat used for protection from injury in a car, bus, or truck crash.

Circumcision - Surgery to take off the loose skin around the top of a baby boy's penis.

Colostrum - The thin, yellowish liquid that comes out of a woman's nipples during pregnancy and the first few days after birth.

Conception - The beginning of a baby's growth, when the mother's egg unites with the father's sperm.

Condom - A rubber or latex tube with a closed end that is put on a man's penis during sex to prevent pregnancy and diseases that can be passed during sex.

Constipation - When bowel movements are very hard and do not come regularly.

Contractions - The tightening and relaxing of the muscle of your uterus.

Development - The ways in which the baby's body grows and the mind learns.

Diarrhea - Bowel movements that are very soft and watery and come more often than usual.

Digestion - The changing of your food in your mouth, stomach, and intestines for use by your body.

Dilation - The stretching open of the mouth of the womb so the baby can be born.

Discharge - Liquid that comes out of your body, like blood or mucus from your vagina.

Drop - The sinking of the unborn baby down into the pelvis before birth begins.

Drugs - Many kinds of things that affect your body or feelings. May be medicines, or substances like alcohol, tobacco, or illegal (street) drugs.

Embryo - Name for a tiny unborn baby during the first eight weeks of its growth.

Engagement - The sinking (dropping) of the baby down into the pelvis before birth.

Engorgement - Hard and painful breasts when milk is starting to be produced.

Episiotomy - A cut made in the skin around the vagina to widen the opening and help the baby to be born.

Family physician or practitioner - A doctor who takes care of the health of people of all ages.

Family planning - Controlling the number of children in the family, and getting pregnant when a person or couple chooses. A birth control method is used so you do not get pregnant from having sex.

Fetal monitoring - A machine that tells how the unborn baby's heart is beating. Used to check the baby's health inside the uterus.

Fetus - The unborn baby, from 8 weeks to birth at about 40 weeks.

Fiber - A substance in foods that helps bowel movements be soft and come regularly.

Formula - Special milk for bottle-feeding. Made to be much like breast milk.

Genetic counseling - Help for people with health problems that may be passed down to their children.

Genetic defects - Health problems that are passed down from parent to child to grandchild through genetic matter in the cells.

Genitals - A boy's penis and girl's vulva.

Gestational Diabetes - A type of diabetes that happens during pregnancy and can cause problems for mother and baby if not found and controlled. Most women are tested at about 26 weeks.

Health care provider - A person trained to take care of people's health and illness (nurses, doctors, nurse-midwives).

Heartburn - A burning feeling in your chest caused by liquid from your stomach going up into the tube from your mouth.

Hemorrhoids - Veins at your anus (opening where bowel movements come out) that get swollen and feel itchy or painful.

Hormones - Substances made by organs in the body that control how it works and feels.

Infection - A sore or illness caused by germs that harm your body.

Iron - A mineral in foods that helps your blood carry oxygen to your baby's body.

Labor - The work your uterus does to open the cervix and push your baby out through the birth canal.

Lactation Specialist - A nurse with special knowledge about breastfeeding (lactation).

Medication - Drugs (medicines) that a doctor prescribes for you or that you can buy at a drug store.

Menstrual period - The blood that flows from a woman's vagina every month.

Midwife - A person who helps women have their babies. Not a doctor.

Miscarriage - Delivery of a baby who is born too early to live or who was ill inside the uterus (spontaneous abortion).

Morning sickness - Name for feeling of nausea and vomiting (being sick to your stomach) in the first few months of pregnancy.

Mucus plug - The thick blob that fills the cervix during pregnancy.

Multiple pregnancy - Twins, triplets, or more babies born at the same time.

Neonatal Intensive Care Unit- The hospital nursery for preterm infants or those with serious medical problems.

Non-aspirin pain reliever - Acetaminophen, a drug better than aspirin for children with pain or fever. "Tylenol" is one common brand.

Nurse-practitioner - A nurse with special training to do some things a doctor usually does.

Nursing - Another word for breastfeeding.

Nutrients - Things in foods that keep you healthy.

Obstetrician-Gynecologist - A doctor who takes care of women's health. An **obstetrician** specializes in prenatal care and delivery of babies. A **gynecologist** specializes in the health of women's uterus and sex organs.

Pelvis - Your hip bones between which your uterus sits. Your vagina (birth canal) goes through a wide opening in these bones.

Pediatrician - A doctor who takes care of children's health.

Pelvic exam - A way for your doctor or nurse-midwife to check your vagina and uterus by pressing on your belly, reaching up inside your vagina, and looking inside.

Perineum - The skin and muscles around the opening of the vagina.

Period - A short name for menstrual period.

Placenta - The organ that connects the mother's body with her fetus. It moves food and oxygen from the mother's blood to the unborn baby's blood.

Pregnancy - The nine months when a woman has a baby growing inside her uterus.

Pregnancy-induced hypertension (PIH) - High blood pressure during pregnancy. May lead to preeclampsia if not treated.

Preterm - A baby born early, before 37 weeks of growth (premature).

Prenatal - Nine-month period when a baby is growing in the mother.

Prescription - An order for medicine from your doctor.

Protein - Substances in food that make your body grow well and work properly.

Sexually-transmitted disease (STD) - A disease passed from one person to another when they have sex.

Spinal cord - The main nerve in the body that goes up the middle of the spine or backbone. It connects the brain to the rest of the body.

Stools - Another term for bowel movements.

Support system - The people in your life or community who help you in times of need.

Swaddling - Wrapping a newborn baby snugly in a thin blanket; comforting.

Symptoms - Changes in your body or how you feel (like pain, itching, or bleeding). These help a doctor or nurse-midwife know what health problem you have.

Trimester - A three-month period. The nine months of pregnancy are divided into three trimesters.

Ultrasound - Special test used to see how your unborn baby is growing. Shows as an image on a screen or photograph.

Umbilical cord - The long tube that attaches the placenta to the unborn baby's body at the navel or "belly button." It carries food and oxygen from the mother's body and wastes from the baby's body. ·

Uterus - The womb, the organ in which an unborn baby grows.

Vaccine - Substance given to immunize against disease.

Vagina - The opening in a woman's body where menstrual bleeding comes out and a man puts his penis during sex. Also the birth canal through which a baby is born.

Vaginal birth - The natural type of birth, in which the baby passes through the cervix and vagina.

Varicose veins - Blue, swollen veins that itch or ache. Often appear in the legs during pregnancy.

VBAC - A short word for Vaginal Birth After a Cesarean birth.

Index: Where to find what you want to know